NEVER A VISCOUNT

SHERI HUMPHREYS

NEVER A VISCOUNT

ISBN 978-1-7332586-3-0 (ebook)
ISBN 978-1-7332586-4-7 (paperback)

Cover design by Christopher Keeslar

❀ Created with Vellum

DANGEROUS SECRETS

A killer is stalking Peter Jennett, Viscount Easterbrook. His cousin's home in the Lake District village of Buttermere seems the perfect place to hide—until Peter is shot and left for dead. His last conscious thought is to hide his identity and confuse his assassin. Forced into the care of a local nurse, the last thing he expects is to discover a woman who makes him wish he were the simple man he pretends to be.

Nurse Anne Albright has never been attracted to a patient, but Peter Matthews, an estate manager wounded by a poacher's errant shot, is special and captures her heart. Then she discovers his secrets, and one is so huge, so personal and so hurtful, she can't forgive him. She'll force herself to nurse him even as he ignores the truth and places a target on his back, and as he helps her face truths of her own.

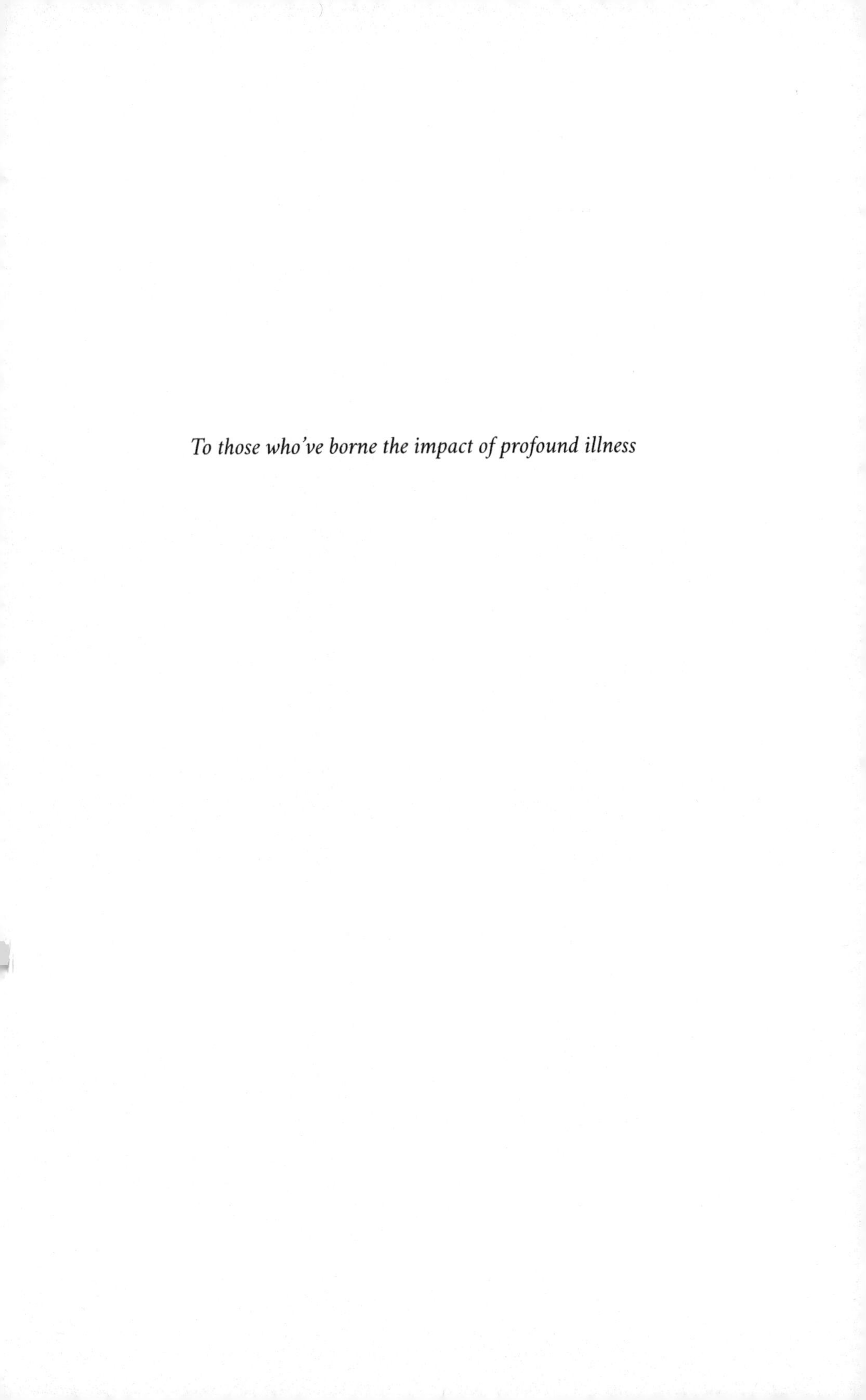

To those who've borne the impact of profound illness

NEVER A VISCOUNT

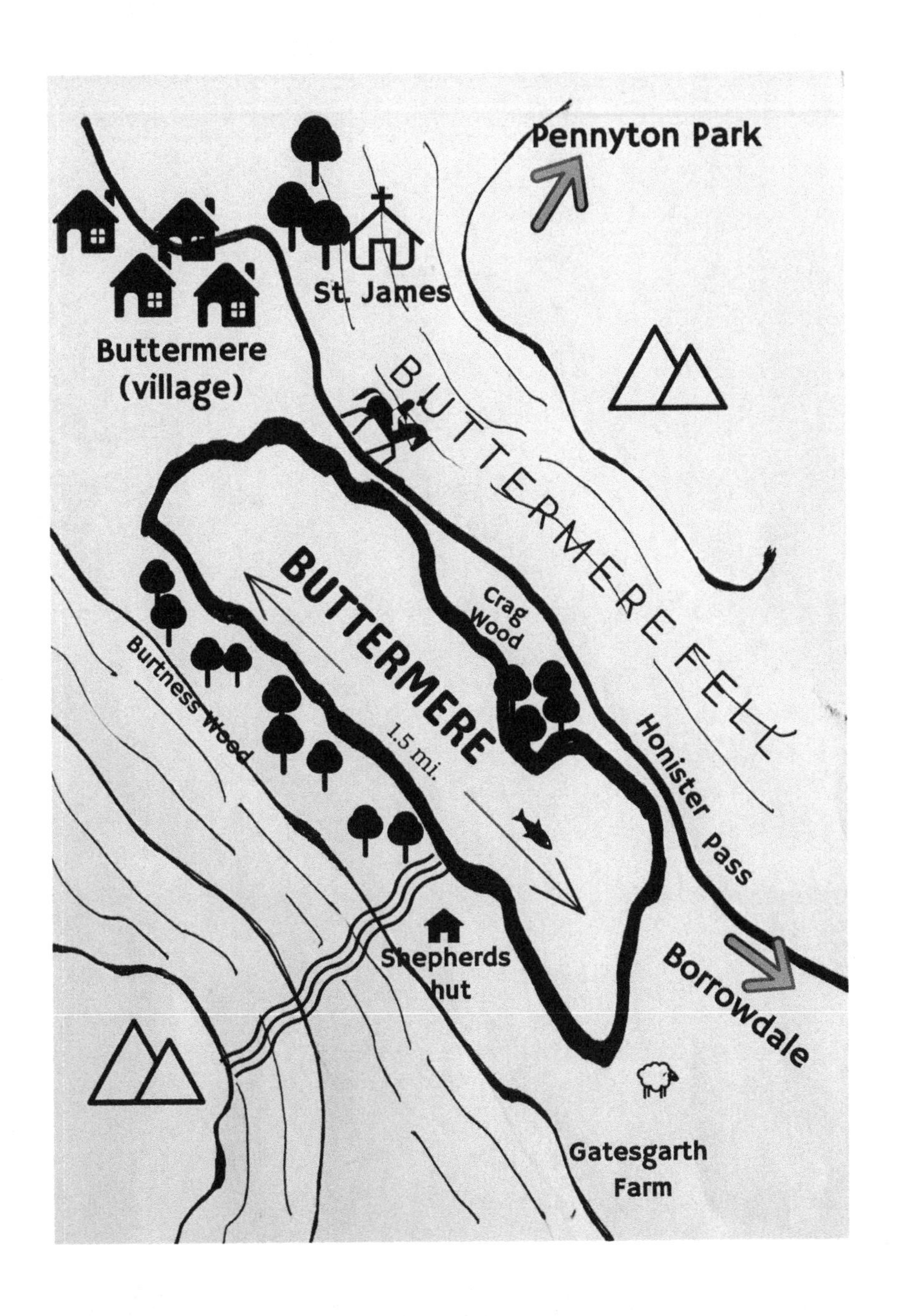
Pennyton Park
St. James
Buttermere
(village)
BUTTERMERE FELL
BUTTERMERE
Crag
Wood
Burtness Wood
1.5 mi.
Honister Pass
Borrowdale
Shepherds
hut
Gatesgarth
Farm

CHAPTER ONE

June 19, 1856

The crack of a rifle split the late afternoon air and a blow hit Peter's back like the hammer of God. The world went sideways and he lost the reins. He grabbed at Red's mane, fisted air, and slammed into the dirt.

Time slipped past in a nauseating whirl before comprehension poked through the muddle. He lay on the road to Buttermere, an exposed puddle of hurt, unable to move. He heard Red grazing. Smelled dirt and blood, and a tinny taste filled his mouth. Inside his head, a throb tolled a warning: *Get up! Get up!*

Fear filled his chest and pinned his back to the ground. His assailant could be approaching to finish the job. He tried to get his hand on the pistol concealed in his coat. Was this how he was to meet his end, like a fly swatted from Red's rump, alone and helpless and not knowing who was trying to kill him? It had to be someone from his closed colliery. He hadn't thought his pursuer would find him in the tiny Lake District village where his cousin Arthur lived. But they had.

Peter strained for his pocket pistol. With a grunt and a last spurt of energy, his fingertips brushed the smooth walnut grip. He tugged the weapon free and rested it on his chest. *Ah, better.* The impending doom drained away. Funny, how comfortable the hard road felt now. Almost cozy....

Something jolted him awake. His gun, snatched from his hand. A big man, his voice too soft to overcome the buzzing in Peter's ears. Was it the shooter, here to finish him off? Every nerve sprang to panicked life.

The man pulled him into a sitting position, and pain burst both from Peter's head and back like an ax had cleaved them open. He strained to get away, but his arms and legs seemed disconnected.

"Bloody hell. Hold still. I'm trying to help you."

The desperate voice, and the intent, penetrated. Relief flooded Peter. This was not his shooter.

With a curse, the man heaved Peter up. The world tilted, receded, rushed back, and a tide of nausea rose. Peter clenched his hands, pressed his palms against the rough hardness beneath him. A wagon bed.

"Red!" Peter pushed his horse's name out.

"I've got him," his rescuer replied. "I've got both of you. Hold on."

The wagon jerked and moved. The jouncing sent white-hot knives stabbing into Peter's back and hobnailed boots stomping his brains.

At last his Good Samaritan pulled up. Peter was cold. Much colder than a June afternoon should warrant, and his eyes wouldn't focus. There came more speaking, more people, more lifting and carrying. He heard a commanding masculine voice that was strangely reassuring, even though the words were not.

Hemorrhage. Surgery. Chloroform. Concussion.

Last, before the pain and the world drifted away, gentle hands and the smell of roses.

~

Peter opened his eyes. Alarm clenched every getaway muscle, then pain speared his back and memories flooded his mind: the road from Borrowdale, the last leg of his unannounced visit to Buttermere and his cousin Arthur. A gunshot.

This time, the person trying to kill him had come close to succeeding.

He was in a bed. Shifting, he moved his arms and legs, and the Devil's pitchfork speared his right upper back and shoulder. Peter cursed. Steel bands cinched his breath from his chest, tight enough to crush lungs, ribs...and denial. This was no mistake, nor were the supposed accidents in London.

Nearby, a woman stood before a corner easy chair where she'd apparently sat and watched him. She crossed the few steps to his bedside, took his wrist, and pressed light fingers to his pulse. He caught the scent of fresh roses, and memories of her fragrance and gentle touch glided through his mind. His tension ebbed.

She had light brown eyes and rich red hair. Peter had never compared eyes to amber or honey, or hair to cinnabar, but those came to mind now.

"Easy," the woman said. "You've been shot."

He knew that, but the word, spoken aloud, gave Peter a little jolt. He gazed around the room. It was tiny, nothing more than clean and serviceable, but out the window he could see sky and trees and a hydrangea bush with blue flowers. His uppermost blanket was glorious art, and he imagined loving hands knitting the bright roses that burst in many-colored splendor from their bed of navy yarn.

He tried to speak but had to stop and swallow. "Where am I?"

His voice sounded as raspy as it felt.

"Mr. Edwin Carter's surgery. You were found yesterday on the road outside the village. You were shot in the back, and your head took a nasty crack when you came off your horse. It's lucky you were nearby. There's not another surgeon or apothecary or physician in Loweswater or Buttermere parishes."

The woman's voice, level and quiet, made Peter wonder how many gunshot victims she'd looked after. Despite her easy tone, he'd wager there hadn't been many in this remote area.

"Who—?" Further words stuck in his parched throat. He coughed, and fire ripped from his back through his chest.

"Here. You need water."

She held a cup in one hand, slipped her other arm under his head and raised it.

His first cautious sip made Peter eager for more. He took a couple thirsty swallows, coughed, and couldn't quite suppress his moan. He paused then tried again, drinking more slowly.

"When you're ready, there's soup on the stove. Food and drink will help your body replenish the blood you lost."

He made a sound of acknowledgement and drank more, then pressed his head against the woman's supporting arm. She eased him back to the pillow without causing a blast of pain. His throat felt better, like he might be able to speak without the words sticking.

"Who are you?"

"Miss Anne Albright. I'm a nurse."

His chest pain settled, and the pulsing in his skull took command. Peter rubbed his forehead. He'd have to get used to using his left hand, since his right arm rested in a sling. "My head feels like someone's been playing cricket with it."

"You sustained a hematoma and a laceration to your scalp. Mr. Carter sewed up the cut."

Peter's fingers explored his head, lingering over the large, tender lump and the silk ligatures. "I'm in Buttermere?"

"Yes. And it's my turn to ask: Who are you?"

Peter hesitated. He'd come from London, watched behind him the whole way, and hadn't seen a soul. Honister Pass didn't offer much cover. The shooter must have been at the farthest reach of his rifle, possibly as far as nine hundred yards, so how certain could he be that the man in his sights was Peter and not someone else? Not one hundred percent. Perhaps Peter could throw him off the trail now instead of confirming he'd been hit but not killed. Should he give a false name? He could ask that his identity be kept secret, but could he trust there'd be no mistakes? News about the man found shot on the road must already be circulating.

"Sir?" the woman repeated. "What is your name? Do you have family in the area?"

"My name is Peter…" What should he do? His cousin Arthur,

rector of Buttermere Parish, lived here. That's why he'd come. But would his presence place Arthur and his family in danger?

His godfather lived in the vicinity, too. The sheer size of Kenton's estate and its many servants would provide protection, but the thought of moving there now, when he was hurting and weak… He needed time. Time to heal. Time to think. And for the foreseeable future, he wasn't able to leave Buttermere Parish.

"Peter." The woman raised her eyebrows. "Peterrrr…"

"Matthews," Peter said, adding a belated *s* to his middle name.

"What brings you to Cumberland, Mr. Matthews?"

Coughing had doubled the pounding in Peter's head. He wished he could sink back into the hazy oblivion in which he'd passed the night and escape the torturous throb, but his brain was awake. Perhaps the distraction of thinking up lies would help.

"I planned to visit a horse breeder in Carlisle. I thought taking an extra couple of days to detour through the lake country would be pleasant."

"I can post a letter to him. Let him know what's happened."

"You needn't bother. He doesn't know when to expect me, so he has no reason to worry."

"Should I write to your family, then?"

"My parents and fiancée are dead."

Peter hadn't intended to share that, but the words just flowed out. This current helpless, cavernous emptiness wasn't all that different from his anguish on the night of the carriage accident. Last night, lying on the ground with the world draining away, he'd faced death just as he had three years ago. Mother, Father, and Louisa, the coachman and footman, all dead and only him alive, diving again and again into the dark, storm-tossed water where pitched segments of the collapsed bridge.

The nurse's hand, nails trimmed and clean, came to rest on his forearm. "I'm sorry, Mr. Matthews."

Her eyes were steady and sincere, and their warmth eased the emptiness a bit. Peter released a gusty sigh and said, "No need to contact anyone just yet. I'll…write my employer in a few days." He wasn't sure who he'd write, actually. Henry Nickerson, his man of business, he supposed, or perhaps Will Aycock, Treewick Hall's estate manager. Good God, his *head*. "Is there anything that might help this pain?"

The nurse's milky skin flushed. She really was quite pretty. "Let me give you a dose of laudanum. It will make you more comfortable."

He hadn't meant to embarrass her, to make her think she hadn't attended him properly. He swallowed the medicine, not even caring it tasted vile. The little crease between her brows made him want to reassure her he'd not suggested neglect. Perhaps continuing their conversation would settle her mind.

"I manage an estate," he offered. He'd always been involved in the running of his properties, and he knew enough to pass for a man who held such a position.

Instead of smoothing, the crease between her eyes deepened. "Do you work for a nobleman, then?"

"Viscount Easterbrook." Easiest to use his own title and estate. "I manage Treewick Hall. It's Easterbrook's family seat, in North Yorkshire."

Something in her expression shifted, giving her a wary look. Curious, too.

"Is he…difficult to work for?"

"Not difficult at all. I'm fond of the fellow."

Her face eased, almost as if she were relieved. "That's good. You should rest and let the laudanum work. I'll dish up some soup in a few minutes. You need nourishment, and you seem to be tolerating water. Call if you need me. The kitchen's close by."

She left. Peter wished he'd thought to ask about Red. He'd ask when she returned.

Oh, his *head*. Wondering whether his brains were about to explode was distracting, but he had to stay alert. Then his stomach flipped as he realized a sharp mind would be of little help. He was incapacitated and would be for some time. His gaze landed on the wall hook that held his trousers. No coat or shirt, they'd have been bloody and torn. His boots rested on the floor below the trousers, his saddlebags alongside. Was his pistol there? It might be wiser to tell the truth, so those around him could be on guard, but knowing his attacker looked for Lord Easterbrook, not Peter Matthews, estate manager, gave him some little increase of security.

Didn't it?

Miss Albright. He'd learn more from her when she returned.

CHAPTER TWO

Anne left the convalescent room. The small chamber didn't get much use. On the rare occasion Edwin had a patient who couldn't be moved or didn't have family to tend an invalid at home, the person was cared for here. The house was both business and home for Edwin, with the surgery situated in front, and the kitchen, small dining room, and sitting room in the back. The bedrooms, all empty save one, were upstairs.

In the kitchen, Anne found Margaret Pettigrew, Edwin's cook-housekeeper, mixing scones and singing. Her deceased husband had been a merchant sailor, and she often sang sea shanties while she worked—even the bawdy ones, which made Anne laugh. The rich smell of beef barley soup permeated the warm, range-heated air, and Anne's stomach rumbled. She clapped a hand to her middle.

"He's awake," she said, interrupting a verse about a skipper's daughter who gave a bit more than she ought. "And I think able to eat soup."

Mrs. Pettigrew's brows rose. "Awake? Is the poor man talking? Did he tell you who he is? What he's doing here?"

The stranger had arrived insensible and nameless. Their only clues to what manner of man he was were his full money bag and a well-bred horse.

"His name is Peter Matthews."

The cook nodded and ladled soup into a bowl as Anne relayed what little else she'd learned about him. "It's a shame he has no friends or family nearby."

Anne took the bowl, spoon, and napkin Mrs. Pettigrew offered and placed them on a serving tray. "I didn't ask him about being shot. I thought it best to leave those questions for the constable." After sustaining a concussion, losing a substantial amount of blood, and having surgery, he'd done well to talk as much as he had. Right now, nourishment would help most. He needed food and more liquids in him.

"It makes me shudder to think he was shot right outside the village," Mrs. Pettigrew said. "If it was a highwayman or the mistake of a poacher, it could've happened to any of us!"

The back door opened, and Michael Elmore entered toting a bucket of coal. The thirteen-year-old boy worked in the house before and after school, doing whatever chores Mrs. Pettigrew asked. An eager look came over his face when he saw Anne, and he said, "Is he awake?"

"Yes. You can let Constable Weaver know, but tell him he's not to come for an hour. The man needs to eat before he's questioned."

"Yes, ma'am." Michael spilled coal into the bin beside the stove and dashed out the door.

Mrs. Pettigrew's gaze swept to the ceiling. "Lad's been driving me barmy asking about him."

The stranger intrigued Anne as well, but in a very different way. Yesterday, after his surgery, she'd washed the unconscious Mr. Matthews's face, hands, and back, and she had done her best to remove the blood from his thick black hair. As unfitting as it was to admire his handsome looks and admirable physique, she couldn't stop herself; unaccustomed awareness had assailed her when she slid a bandage roll under his back and around his chest. Once she'd had the wrap complete and tied in place, she'd smoothed the blankets and positioned his relaxed arm along his side, atop the cover, but the rugged strength of his hand kept drawing her eyes. For just a moment she'd rested her palm on the back of his hand. An urge to lace their fingers together overcame her, and she'd curled her fingertips the tiniest bit, wondering how it would feel to be touched by that very masculine, blunt-fingered hand....

She'd snatched her hand away then, horrified, and hurried to the corner chair. Afterward, she'd managed to confine her thoughts to those appropriate for a nurse observing her patient—but then he'd woke and conversed with her, which had fueled her fascination to an even greater height. Self-confident, intelligent, capable... She marveled at his composure after being shot. All those traits, combined with his male beauty, made him wholly remarkable here in the simple environs of Buttermere Parish. Who was he? A war veteran, a man accustomed to danger?

The bell on the surgery's front door tinkled, the door slammed, and Anne stopped daydreaming. She knew that tread.

Edwin.

He entered the kitchen, and his gaze went from the humming and busy Mrs. Pettigrew, to the soup bowl on the tray, then to Anne. "Looks like he's awake."

"His name is Peter Matthews. He was on a business trip and a holiday, and he has no one in the area. He drank some water and took a dose of laudanum. No bleeding, no confusion, no vomiting."

"Good. I worried about his head, given how long he stayed semiconscious. Any fever?" Edwin smoothed back his disheveled light brown hair and adjusted his spectacles as he spoke. His beard, fuller than the current fashion, made him seem older than the thirty-four years Anne knew him to be. He was a good man, an accomplished surgeon they were all grateful to have in the area. He'd be a wonderful father and husband—if he ever made time to find the right woman as Anne so frequently urged him to do.

"No fever."

Edwin gave a nod and headed toward the convalescent room. Anne followed with the soup and tea.

Dragging a wooden chair away from the wall, Edwin set it near their patient and sat.

The patient looked up and said, "You must be Mr. Carter."

"I am. Edwin Carter, surgeon and apothecary. You look like Miss Albright has worked her usual magic. Feeling better, are you, Mr. Matthews?"

"Yes." The man began to make stretching motions, tilting his head to the side and moving his uninjured shoulder. "Uuuuuungh." He stilled then clamped his teeth through a deep breath. "Better until I moved," he admitted, acknowledging his stupidity. "I gather you performed the surgery. What are my injuries?"

"You took a rifle shot to your scapula, the right upper back. The bone stopped the Minié ball but sustained fractures. I removed a few bone splinters when I extracted the slug. There's nothing more to do for your shoulder but keep your arm in a sling. It should mend."

Edwin stood, retrieved the bullet from the dresser, and offered the once conical but now misshapen lump to Mr. Matthews. Anne had cleaned it. Matthews took the Minié and examined it the way he might a puzzle. It must feel strange to him, holding the crumpled chunk of lead that might have ended his life.

Edwin resumed his seat. "By the time Gilbert Marshall found you and got you here, you'd bled a fair amount. Miss Albright administered chloroform, and I located and removed the ball."

"Is Marshall a big man? I remember someone lifting me."

"That's him. His sheep farm is nearby."

Matthews fisted the bullet and returned his gaze to Edwin. "Lucky for me. Did he hear the shot? See anyone?"

"He heard the shot but didn't see a soul. Your money was still on you, so it wasn't a highwayman unless he scrupled not to shoot two men in pursuit of it. I hate to think a poacher shot you by accident and was so afraid of the consequences he left you for dead. . . ." Edwin shook his head. "That kind of thing just doesn't happen here. Perhaps the constable will have more information. I told him he could come by today."

The two men sat silently for a moment, then Edwin rubbed his fingers over his beard and continued.

"So, I irrigated your wound and closed it with ligature. Sutured the laceration on your scalp, too. Marshall thought you'd been unconscious, and you talked nonsense for a while after you got here. I'm certain you have a concussion. Time will tell how bad the brain bruising is, but you can expect dizziness and nausea and a headache that could last for days. Confusion. Memory loss. Let Miss Albright or myself know whatever bothers you, but given any unforeseen complications your recovery from the head injury should be otherwise unremarkable." Edwin paused then mentioned what Anne knew was the unnerving part. "The complication of wound infection is more likely, and worrisome. We'll have to wait and see."

Both men wore grave expressions. Everyone had acquaintances and family who'd died from infection.

"I'm grateful for all you've done," Matthews said at last. "Thank you. Both of you," he added, looking at Anne. "I didn't know nurses administered chloroform."

"Usually they don't, but Mr. Carter trained me. In addition to working here in the surgery, I make home visits to change bandages and keep watch on healing wounds, that sort of thing. Some families need daily help for one reason or another. I also assist my mother whenever she needs an extra pair of hands. She's the midwife."

"Annie, you don't acknowledge your abilities as you should!" Edwin looked at Matthews and shook his head. "She was still a child when she started apprenticing with her mother. When I settled here Annie was fourteen, had already delivered several babies, and had acquired a good measure of the knowledge, skill, and experience a midwife needs. She kept coming by, asking if she could study my medical books and begging to help me in the surgery. Once I agreed, she stopped working with her mother and trained under me instead. I can't imagine a better assistant."

"Sounds like I was fortunate to be shot in this parish," Matthews joked.

Edwin chuckled. "You could have done worse. We're all fortunate to have Anne. When I'm gone making home visits, which is most days, Anne will be here keeping watch." He stood and turned to her. "We should order more thorn-apple. Michael says Tim's been wheezing. He hasn't been bad enough to need a treatment, but something's exacerbating his asthma and our supply is getting low."

Anne nodded. Sometimes the younger Elmore's breathing became so restricted, thorn-apple was the only thing that helped. "I'll do a quick inventory and get our order in the mail."

"First thing tomorrow will be fine," Edwin said. "Yesterday was a long day and you started early this morning. You get on home after Mr. Matthews eats his soup."

Anne nodded. "All right."

At the door, Edwin half turned. "I'll be checking on you," he assured their patient, "but if you need me during the night, don't hesitate to ring. I'm a light sleeper when there's a patient in the house."

He left then, and Anne turned her attention back to Mr. Matthews.

"Let's get some nourishment in you." Soup in hand, she sat in the chair Edwin had vacated. "Sitting up will be painful, so today I'll feed you. Tomorrow you can sit up and drink your soup from a mug."

Matthews grunted. He set the Minié ball atop the small bedside table on his left and said, "I want to sit up today."

Before she could set the bowl down, he began to rise. Effort and pain creased his face, and Anne almost dropped the soup in her hurry to place it on the table. Moving to support his back, and careful to avoid his wound, she pulled him forward the last bit as he groaned. Then he sat, grimacing and breathing hard, clutching his head.

"Queen Victoria's cat. This might *not* be such a good idea." He closed his eyes and didn't resist when Anne eased him back until he once again lay flat. Body stretched full-length, his feet stuck off the end of the small bed.

"You're weak. You'll feel better after you eat," Anne promised. She rearranged the pillows so his head and shoulders were elevated, spread a napkin under his chin, and offered him a spoonful of soup.

After the first swallow, his eyebrows rose. "Mmm." He glanced at her, gave a small nod, and returned his attention to eating.

They were quiet as he accepted spoonfuls. He didn't hold up a staying hand until he'd consumed two-thirds of the bowl, and Anne was satisfied with that.

He plucked the napkin from his chest, swiped at his mouth, and tossed the linen to his abdomen. "I hate feeling helpless."

"Each day will be easier," she said, hoping it would be true. It was encouraging that he had an appetite. "You have a strong constitution. What you've already come through proves that." She stood and pointed near the head of the bed. "There's a bell on that table. Ring if you need anything. Mr. Carter will hear."

Matthews frowned. "The two of you are betrothed?"

That question—and the man's look—took her aback. Tension bloomed in Anne's stomach like yellow dandelions after rain and sunshine. There was nothing romantic between her and Edwin, in spite of how sensible and expected those who knew them would consider such a match. They had much more in common than she and Andrew Snow, who *was* courting her, and who had recently proposed, in fact. But why would *Mr. Matthews* think that? Also, he sounded as if he didn't like the idea. His eyes almost seemed accusing. Why? He didn't know them. And why should she care if he cared?

"No. What made you think that?"

The lines on Matthews's forehead deepened. "He called you Annie."

Anne's face burned. The dandelions turned to white, feathery seed-head tufts, flew apart, and bashed around in her stomach. "Mr. Carter is a good friend. When we're private we use our first names. Using mine in front of you was a lapse of the tongue is all. We're not promised."

Edwin was the brother she'd never had; it was that simple. Her possible future with Andrew Snow was another matter. She was twenty-four years old, had never been in love, and more than anything, as foolish as it seemed, wanted to love the man she married. Why wasn't her fondness of Andrew growing into something more passionate? Something like what happened now as Mr. Matthews considered her, a sudden awareness of her femininity that made

Anne's skin sensitive, made her feel the fabric of her clothing rubbing and pressing. Could he tell how he affected her, and how new it all was? Anne's heart filled her chest and confusion filled her mind. What was she to do about these improper, womanly feelings?

His arm moved; he offered the napkin. She reached out, grasped the linen, and his finger grazed hers. A quiver raced up her arm and danced over her shoulders. She pulled the fabric from his grasp, stood, picked up the tray, and stepped away.

Breathed.

His forehead smoothed, and her heart shrank to its normal size.

"Try to sleep," she said after a moment. "I'll see you tomorrow."

She thought he was going to smile, but he didn't, and every step home she wished she could turn back and be the one to watch over him.

CHAPTER THREE

A noise woke Peter. He'd drifted off to sleep with food in his belly and the laudanum damping his pain down to a tolerable level, but judging by the angle of the late afternoon sunshine slanting through the nearby window he hadn't slept long. He blinked, sharpening the bleary image of a man standing in his room.

"How do you do, Mr. Matthews," the man said. "I'm Constable Thomas Weaver. I apologize for waking you, but I was told this would be a good time for us to talk."

"You're not disturbing me," Peter assured him. "Have a seat." This was as good a time as any, and his bonfire of a headache had died to glowing coals.

The constable closed the door, removed his hat, and sat on the same chair Carter and Miss Albright had used.

"My name's not Matthews," Peter began. "I'm Viscount Easterbrook, Peter Jennett."

Weaver's eyebrows shot up and he cocked his head. "Are you, now? I presume Arthur Jennett is a relative?"

"My cousin."

Weaver leaned back and crossed his arms. "I'm guessing the rector doesn't know you're here?"

"Not yet. I'd appreciate you letting him know."

"You can tell him yourself. Not an hour ago he told me he intends to stop by before heading home, to pay his respects to the wounded stranger."

The news swept gladness through Peter. There was no one he'd rather see. "He's not going to like that I chose to be incognito, but I felt I had to."

Weaver shifted forward, placed elbows on thighs and held his hat between his knees. "And why's that, my lord?"

"To protect Arthur and his family. Yesterday was the third time someone's tried to kill me. Last month there were two attempts in London. After the second, I wanted to hide away. I left town suddenly, at night, without informing anyone." Even his valet and butler didn't know where he was. He'd left them notes, slipped out, and walked to the stable.

"Buttermere is small and remote," he continued, looking meaningfully at the constable, "and I thought Arthur's home would be the perfect place to disappear while I figured out what to do." He'd thought he'd be safe, thought it was somewhere he could relax and breathe and think. How in the hell had the shooter followed him? "It's a long way for a man to track and not be seen. And I'd expected anyone searching for me to think I'd gone to my country estate!"

"You think the gunman might yet be convinced he shot the wrong man?"

He had a keen mind, this constable. "Exactly. That's why I didn't want to give my name or ask for my cousin. It was a hasty decision, but I don't regret it. As Mr. Matthews, I don't have to worry about my presence somehow endangering Arthur and his family—assuming we can keep up the pretense."

Weaver leaned back against his chair and tapped the brim of his hat on his knee. "If this was intentional, then, in spite of the precautions you took, and are taking, someone *did* follow. Who's trying to kill you? Do you know?"

Peter sighed. "It's complicated. I've an entire village in Yorkshire angry with me. I'm partner in a colliery there, and I closed the mine, which left the majority of residents out of work. I think one or two laborers are furious enough to do me harm. My business partner isn't too happy with me, either."

"Why did you close the mine?" Weaver asked. "Is the coal depleted?"

"There's still a large deposit, but the easily accessible coal is gone. Workers have to go deeper. The danger has increased to a degree I can't justify sending men down there. Collapse and lack of ventilation are both of significant concern."

"Any other sources of livelihood in the area?"

"Not many. The colliery supports most of Cliff Gate. I've hired an engineer, a graduate of the new Government School of Mines. He's there, evaluating. I hope he'll find a solution and the closure will be temporary. I couldn't keep paying all of them a full wage, though, as much as I might wish to. One would hope their lives would be worth more than..." He trailed off.

Weaver nodded slowly. One corner of his mouth thinned, and one eye narrowed. "Those miners might be angry, but how would your death help them?"

"My partner opposed the shutdown. Perhaps someone's anger or desire for revenge has overcome common sense and they think he and my heir might reopen the mine—though they couldn't be sure of that. But no one else has motive to kill me!" Peter paused, not quite sure of his words. Hardesty, maybe. His partner. He'd racked his brain, and there was no one else. Not unless—

No.

"If the laborers are that determined to work the mine, why not let them? They know the risk and they accept it. It's part of being a collier."

Exactly what Hardesty had argued. "I understand they don't object to the risk. But the deeper we go, the higher the probability of gas explosion or collapse. If such a disaster happened... I can't even imagine. I'd feel responsible. I'm hoping the engineer will offer strategies to increase safety." Peter shrugged his uninjured shoulder. "But I think I may have made things worse for myself by being kind."

"How's that?" Weaver asked, settling back in his chair and looking a tiny bit skeptical. Peter didn't blame him.

"We only hire men. None younger than seventeen. The pay is higher than what other owners offer, and I try to keep the conditions far better than at other mines. So these men haven't just lost a job, they've lost the best job they've ever had. And they likely think I should be able to keep paying them full wages, regardless of if the mine is in operation. I can't."

Weaver studied him for a moment. "No?"

"No." Peter shook his head. "But it's not just about the money, which is my point. Many mines go as deep as Bellow Hill. Deeper, even. Those owners are just collecting the profits. But they don't think about what happens if their workers are killed, how those families are left to starve...."

He couldn't help the note of derision in his voice. In all his business dealings, Peter wanted to do more: not just make money for himself, but better the lives of those associated with his concerns. The first time he'd seen how he could improve others' lives, he'd become a devotee. And it was so easy! A little less profit for himself, a little more money in the pockets of his workers and tenants. There was nothing like the feeling when he saw a man's bleak, defeated gaze fill with pride and hope. But kindness in business had its downsides.

Weaver stood, stuck his hands in his pockets, strode to the window and looked out. "So, in your workers' minds—or some of them—you're overcautious and unreasonable. You mentioned your partner. Does he feel the same? Can he withstand the current loss?"

Peter sighed. The last time he'd seen Hardesty, the man was livid about the impending closure and half wages, but he'd apparently gone to Cliff Gate, the village closest to the mine and where most of its laborers lived. In his last letter, George Lawton, the engineer Peter hired, had written that, with the exception of when he went down into the mine, Hardesty was staying at his side, asking questions and pressuring him for solutions and speed, and generally making his life miserable. But didn't that mean he had settled down and accepted that Peter, who held the majority share, wasn't swaying?

"I can't imagine him deciding to murder me." Peter shook his head. Hardesty had a comfortable fortune.

Of course, fortunes could change.

"Perhaps I should see what I can discover about his current financial state." Peter ruminated a moment. "If it *is* Hardesty, he'd hire someone to do the job. Still...I just can't see it."

Weaver nodded, turned, and put his back to the window. "Tell me about the other attempts."

Peter straightened and stared at the ceiling, exhausted; what energy the soup had provided had drained away. He was tired of talking and wanted to rest. If only Arthur would come.

"Three weeks ago I was jostled—tripped—into a busy London street. I was nearly trampled." In fact, a pair harnessed to a curricle had reared over his sprawled body. He'd been right under their uplifted hooves. He still wasn't sure how he'd managed to roll out of the way in time. "I thought that an accident. Then it happened again. The second time I was pushed hard, and it was more luck I wasn't severely injured. I fell against a carriage that was traveling at a good clip. Just missed going under the wheel and sustained a lot of bruising."

He'd had a difficult time wrapping his mind around the events and accepting that they had been intentional, to be honest. But now, with this gunshot being the third near miss...

Weaver dropped into his chair and trained sharp hazel eyes on Peter. "I have an idea. My son is home from the army after losing an arm in the Crimea. He's a good man, still finding his feet. I wonder if he might not be suitable for investigating in Yorkshire?"

Peter considered. The constable had asked thoughtful questions and done more listening than talking. If the son's character resembled the father's, this was a good idea. The constable was right; someone did need to investigate. Writing to his man of business, then waiting while someone appropriate was located, interviewed, and hired, might take weeks. Peter could hire Weaver's son and dispatch him by tomorrow or the day after.

He considered the constable further. The man's mouth had

stretched into a thin-lipped smile, one corner angled higher than the other. His expression, his tilted-forward posture, and his tight jaw gave him a rather intense appearance. He'd take young Weaver's measure and see if it was the same.

"I like your plan," Peter decided. "Have your son come round tomorrow."

Weaver gave a nod and stood. "I'll be keeping a close eye out, but I think you're safe here, *Mr. Matthews*. Strangers stand out, and this surgery is on Buttermere's main road." He secured his bowler and gave the brim a flick. "I'm sorry you're in these circumstances, but they present me with a challenge. And I'm a man who likes a challenge."

Weaver left the door open as he exited, and quiet reigned for a quarter-hour. Then the bell attached to the front door tinkled, and the sound of a long stride crossed the empty waiting room and came down the short hall. Anticipation and relief rose from Peter's core and spilled into every part of his body as Arthur appeared in the doorway.

Joy blasted through Peter. His cousin, however, stopped so abruptly he wobbled. His mouth fell open and he looked stunned, as if he'd slipped on ice and landed hard, and he fought for words.

"Quiet," Peter said in a low voice, waving him over. "Let me explain, Arthur."

His cousin walked to the bed as if *he'd* been shot, tossed his hat on the small table there, and grabbed the chair rail as if he needed something to hold. His eyebrows snapped together as he said, "*You're* the man found shot? Why didn't you send for me? Why doesn't anyone know who you are?" He paused a beat. "Are you all right?"

Peter offered his hand, and the two gripped hard. Arthur sat and scooted the chair as close to the bed as it would go, gave him a stern look and said, "Well? Are you all right?"

"I was lucky. My shoulder blade stopped the bullet."

"But why didn't you send word? To walk in and find you like this..."

"I know. I'm sorry. Everything happened fast."

Arthur swept back the hair hanging over his forehead, hair so like

Peter's own. Their fathers had been brothers, and Peter and Arthur both had black locks, the same tall, lean build, and the aquiline nose displayed by generations of Jennetts in family portraits. Arthur wore clergyman's garb now: a white shirt with stand-up clerical collar, a black waistcoat that buttoned high on the chest to create a notch at the base of the throat, and a long black coat.

Eyes cast down, Arthur exhaled through pursed lips, his cheeks puffing out, and Peter's heart flopped. By not notifying his cousin right away, he'd hurt and confused him.

"I'm sorry," he repeated, not knowing what else to say. His back and head pain were building; each throb seemed more intense than the last. Talking to Constable Weaver had exhausted him, but Arthur waited and he didn't want to let his cousin down any further. "I need a dose of laudanum. Could you ring the bell?"

Arthur lifted the item from Peter's bedside table and jangled it hard. A moment later, a woman with salt-and-pepper hair and a bright white apron appeared.

"Mr. Jennett," she said with a smile. "How nice to see you. And Mr. Matthews, how do you do? I'm Mrs. Pettigrew. Would you gentlemen like tea?"

"Hello, Mrs. Pettigrew," Arthur said. "Tea would be welcome, and —" He stopped abruptly and cleared his throat. "Mr. Matthews needs pain tonic."

"Mr. Carter said he might. Let me get that first."

The housekeeper went into the treatment room and returned a moment later with Peter's measure of laudanum. Then she retired to the kitchen.

"What's going on?" Arthur asked once they were alone again.

Peter sighed. "Someone wants me dead. It has to be one of the miners at Bellow Hill. He made two previous tries in London. I left. Intended to hide out with you, but somehow the ruffian tracked me down and—"

"Queen Victoria's cat!"

Hearing his cousin utter that unique, irreverent curse made the center of Peter's chest go soft and warm. He and Arthur had devised and started using the phrase as boys, after being punished for saying something much less genteel. From the age of nine, when Arthur's father died and Arthur and his mother came to live at Treewick Hall, until they graduated from university, the two had rarely been apart. For a moment the pain and exhaustion receded, and Peter chuckled.

"Stop laughing," Arthur snapped. "It's not a laughing matter."

"It's just so good to see you."

The two paused and exchanged the affectionate smile they'd shared hundreds of times over the years—smiles that said without words or brotherly embrace how each knew the other's soul. Then Arthur nodded and Peter went on to repeat much of what he'd told Weaver already.

Brows furrowed, his cousin listened, then responded the moment Peter stopped speaking. "Do you really think the shooter doesn't know who you are? He shot you."

"I don't see how he could be certain," Peter replied. "He was a long way behind me or I'd have seen him."

Arthur crossed his arms. "Then he's desperate and probably deranged. I don't like it. I want you safe, in my home."

Aside from the changes maturity had wrought, his cousin's expression looked just as alarmed as it had the day Peter fell from their favorite oak. Then Arthur closed his eyes and dropped his head, and after a huge breath he added, "But if there's a chance your being there would place Belinda and the children in danger..."

He looked up, and Peter saw those same clear gray eyes he'd known all his life—honest, loyal, full of love, and glistening with tears—and Peter nodded. The two men fell into a silent, unspoken agreement.

Mrs. Pettigrew returned and soon had them situated with steaming tea. She handed Peter a mug instead of a teacup, and he found he was able to manage it on his own. "Good for you, Mr. Matthews," she said before exiting.

The comfort of Arthur's presence and the warmth of the tea in his stomach seemed to augment the effect of Peter's laudanum. His cousin seemed lost in thought, though, the frown still carving lines in his brow.

"You should drink that before it goes cold," Peter prompted.

Arthur looked up. "Thank God you weren't killed." His cousin's throat moved in what seemed a hard swallow. "I never think of it, but...have you considered that *I* have a stronger motive to see your toes turned up to the daisies than anyone else in the world?"

Peter paused, embarrassed. He had. Arthur was his heir. If Peter died, his property, wealth, title, *everything* would go to him. But...that was impossible. "If the skunk manages to kill me, don't reopen the mine until it's safe."

Arthur's brow smoothed, and the corners of his mouth angled up. "I promise."

Peter pushed on, meaning to reassure his cousin further. "Tell Belinda to come visit. Or would it seem odd for the rector's wife to call on a stranger? I'd love to see the children, too."

"I could bring them," Arthur agreed. But he massaged his earlobe.

Peter waited. Arthur only tugged at his ear when something discomfited him. Was it about his wife? It was hard to imagine the woman unhappy with Arthur, but in his last two letters, his cousin had expressed concerns. The last time he'd seen them, for Rebecca's christening, Belinda had seemed a contented wife and mother. They'd shared a few days' holiday before the Bishop of Carlisle performed the ceremony.

"I suppose I should tell you."

Peter raised his brows and waited. Arthur would speak when he was ready.

"Belinda and Miss Albright are thought to be half-sisters."

The ground under Peter's feet disappeared. He'd spent a fair amount of time mountaineering, and the worst fall he'd ever taken had been on Monte Rosa. This felt like tumbling down that icy slope all over again: mind whirling, limbs disconnected, heart in his throat. Out of control.

"What?"

"It's generally believed that Anne Albright is my father-in-law's illegitimate daughter. Born ten months after Belinda."

"Arthur. I… What are you saying? Kenton—*James* Kenton—fathered Anne Albright?"

It wasn't possible. He *knew* Kenton. Had known him all his life. Had *looked up* to him all his life. Six years ago, when the living at Buttermere Parish had come available, Peter was the one who recommended Arthur to Kenton. The viscount's patronage had secured Arthur's appointment as rector, though none had anticipated that, two years later, Arthur would marry the man's daughter. And *that* Viscount Kenton had sired an illegitimate daughter? The daughter was Anne Albright, the young woman with competent hands and kind eyes who smelled of roses?

Peter's cousin dragged his hand down his face. "I'm sorry. I first thought of telling you when Belinda and I married, but I decided against it. I knew it would change the way you thought of him."

"'Change the way I thought of him…?" Since Peter's father's death, Kenton had been the man Peter sought when he needed wise counsel. "You're damn right it changes the way I think of him. I've always believed him to be the best of men. Now I discover he's an adulterer?"

Peter shook his head. For a moment it was the day after Louisa's funeral, and he stood alone at his parents' graveside. There were business associates, friends, and family retainers scattered about, but no one intimate. No one that could melt the freezing cold that had seized him the night they died. Arthur had been forced to remain in Cumberland; he and Belinda expected the birth of their first child any day. Arthur's mother, Aunt Esther, was in Scotland and wouldn't arrive in time. Peter sensed every eye upon him, the new Viscount Easterbrook. He'd never felt so alone. Then a strong hand clamped his shoulder: Kenton, standing beside him. His father's best friend from his university days, the man his father had named Peter's godfather. The last time he'd seen Kenton had been the night of Peter's betrothal dinner to Louisa.

"I'm here," Kenton had said, and gave Peter's shoulder a squeeze, warming him and dispelling that aching cold. Peter had seen abject sorrow in his godfather's eyes, too. The man looked tired and pale, the skin around his eyes puffy, and as he stayed by Peter's side through the service and afterwards, remaining at Treewick Hall several days, Peter was never so grateful to not be alone. He knew every one of Kenton's five children and counted each a friend. How could there be a daughter that none spoke of? And how could Anne—he really preferred to think of her by her given name and not as Miss Albright—be that secret daughter?

"You should have told me."

"I'm no scandalmonger. Advising you seemed like sharing dirty secrets, and you didn't need to know. It wouldn't have been right."

Anger chopped through Peter with the brutal thoroughness of a butcher's cleaver. "Of course I needed to know!"

"I understand you're unhappy to discover his name linked to unsavory conduct, but it's my, Belinda and her family's concern."

"And Anne's," Peter muttered. He tried to restrain his displeasure with Arthur. He'd consider the rightness or wrongness of his cousin's decision later. "Kenton supports her, I assume?"

For a moment Arthur didn't answer. His mouth tightened. "You assume wrong. Kenton never admitted to being Miss Albright's father." He let out a hefty sigh. "There's more. Emma Albright, the mother, accused him of rape."

"Rape!" Another burning whirlpool of disbelief spun in Peter's brain. "Kenton wouldn't rape anyone."

Arthur grimaced. "He responded to her accusation by saying something about his being a gentleman, not a defiler of innocent women. But she continued to accuse him. Perhaps it was an ill-advised or bungled attempt to extort money. Kenton never said anything further, and eventually his silence was interpreted to mean he admitted to having congress with the lady—consensual congress. Weaver told me everyone in the village took sides, with most supporting Kenton's claim of innocence. The Albrights believed their daughter. Emma and Anne lived with them, and Emma inherited the house a couple years ago. They live...frugally."

"Rape is a crime!" Peter said, wondering how such an injustice—if true—could go unpunished.

"Kenton's a viscount, and there was no evidence. He'd never be charged."

That was true, Peter realized. What a sad muddle.

Oddly, though he should be thinking about his godfather and not his illegitimately sired nurse, he found himself wondering how the situation had affected Anne. She must believe her mother. How horrible! Not only to be deprived of the loving father every child should have had, but to believe her existence came about through violence.

A groan escaped him. "This kind of scandal's not something people forget."

"No," Arthur agreed. "No one's forgotten. Kenton's here for a few months every year. Each time he arrives, the gossip recirculates. He's not here now, though. Lady Kenton is, but he's gone to Ascot." Peter's cousin rose, retrieved his hat then stepped over and gave Peter's shoulder a comforting squeeze—not unlike the gesture Kenton had made three years ago. Peter placed his hand atop Arthur's, and for the moment he pushed aside thoughts of Kenton's infidelity and just appreciated being with family. The relief of reconnecting with his trustworthy, perfectly loyal cousin was like the first open sky, warm spring day after a harsh winter, and Peter's heart swelled until it felt in danger of bursting from his chest.

After a second encouraging squeeze, Arthur stepped away and secured his low-crowned hat. "I'll keep you in my prayers."

"Thank you," Peter said. And he meant it.

"I'll bring Belinda and the children soon," Arthur said, obviously coming to a decision about the issues of paternity and whether they were enough to stop him. "You want us to pretend we're calling on a wounded traveler? We're to keep up the ruse to your caregivers as well?"

The deception weighed heavy on Peter's conscience. Should he reveal his identity to Carter and Anne? Would Anne feel uncomfortable caring for him if she knew his connection to her supposed father? Worse, might either Carter or Anne slip in the presence of Mrs. Pettigrew or the lad who worked about the place, thus ensuring the information made it to the village?

"I deserve to be stoned, asking you to lie," he said at last, "but I think it safest."

Arthur hesitated then nodded. "I have faith in God that in this instance He'll excuse me. See you tomorrow...Mr. Matthews." He started to leave then paused, stared at the floor a long moment, then lifted his head and drew a deep breath. "There's something else I should tell you. When you see Belinda, you'll find her changed."

His cousin's face had gone grim, and Peter's chest grew tight. "How?" he asked.

"She's lost weight and just picks at her food. The baby sleeps through the night now, yet Belinda's still irritable and short-tempered and sleeps poorly. She seems...unhappy."

"That is concerning," Peter said—somewhat lamely, he knew. He didn't know what else to say. He'd considered Arthur and Belinda the happiest, most deeply in love couple he knew. They'd been his ideal for the perfect marriage, and he'd taken great pleasure in knowing his cousin had found joy in both his work and family.

"She denies anything is wrong," Arthur continued, "but it's been going on for months—since Rebecca's birth. I'm at my wits' end. I demanded she see a physician, but she refused. We argued about it so much that she finally agreed to let Carter examine her, but he couldn't offer an explanation. I don't know what to do."

"I'm sorry," Peter said.

"And I'm sorry to burden you with this, but you'll see for yourself soon enough. I always knew Belinda's privileged upbringing didn't prepare her for life as a clergyman's wife..." Arthur expressed a humorous sound that wasn't quite a laugh and his eyes got misty. "Imagine not only my surprise but my dilemma when we fell in love. The rector's living here is a good one, but it doesn't provide near what Belinda was accustomed to as Kenton's daughter. A modest home, tiny in comparison to her father's estates. A practical wardrobe, with dresses others might admire but not covet, when she was used to the loveliest fashions and finest fabrics." Peter's cousin's mouth flattened;

his smile turning wooden and cheerless. "As much as I loved her, I almost didn't propose. I knew my wife would be expected to do things Belinda had no experience with and never imagined herself doing. She convinced me that she not only could do it, but wanted to. I worry that with the additional work of the baby it's become too much for her."

"I'm sorry, Arthur," Peter repeated, still at a loss for what to say. How had they never discussed this? "I suppose parish duties can be burdensome."

Arthur released a gusty exhale. "Well," he offered, obviously taking control of his feelings. "As much as I hate adding to your worries, it's a relief to talk about this with you. Lately the situation has rested especially heavy on my mind. I've even entertained the far-fetched and utterly ridiculous notion of a renewed attraction between Belinda and Richard Thorpe. He was her first love, and he still works for her father. He always singles her out at church and talks a few minutes. That's how awful it's been, me seeing *that* as a threat."

Peter had twice been introduced to Thorpe by Kenton. He was the man responsible for Kenton's rising reputation in the Steeplechase world. Arthur was correct, though. The idea of Belinda favoring any other man was ridiculous, and even more so was the possibility of her reacting to the austerity of the life of a vicar's wife by attraction to a different man of lesser means.

"I'm glad you told me," Peter said, "but I'm sure you have nothing to worry about."

Arthur nodded, gave him a smile that looked forced, and left.

Peter listened to his cousin's footsteps, the door opening and closing, and then the quiet. This confirmed it. The world had gone topsy-turvy crazy. He massaged the weary tension underlying his forehead and eyes and grappled with the shocking revelations of the past twenty-four hours. Someone had nearly killed him. Arthur's once ideal marriage was in turmoil. And Kenton, the godfather he admired for his analytical mind, his generosity, and his trustworthiness...*no*. He just couldn't believe the rumor. The idea that Kenton could have forced himself upon an unwilling woman was outlandish.

Memories crowded Peter's mind, most of them of his father and Kenton: Kenton's booming laugh after Peter's father told one of his bitingly witty stories. The way Kenton vaulted from the saddle after a stumble and carefully examined his mount's leg. The identical looks of pride on his godfather's and father's faces when Peter graduated from Oxford... And then that kaleidoscope slowed and an especially vivid recollection crowded the others out: his father and Kenton arguing. Their irate voices stuck Peter's feet to the hall floor just outside his father's study.

"Good God, John," he heard Kenton say. "Break free of the old agrarian model. It doesn't work anymore, and you're not your father. It's a new world. A world of industry and invention, a world begging for investment capital. After years of struggling to retain your properties, you've the opportunity to grow your wealth."

Peter had backed against the wall, listening. Those words were exactly what *he* had told his father, himself.

"There's the opportunity to lose it all, too." That had been his father's reply, his father's conservative, certain, I'm-not-about-to-risk-losing-my-assets voice. "My bank account has shrunk more than I like, but I've managed to keep the Easterbrook holdings intact. If I die tomorrow, Peter will inherit the same properties and businesses that my great-grandfather and grandfather and father passed down."

"But will he be able to hold on to them?" Kenton asked. "Not following your example, not the last half of this century, he won't!"

His father had laughed, and gooseflesh broke Peter's skin. The laugh wasn't a warm expression of humor, but a disheartened sound of desperation.

"He doesn't want to oversee the Easterbrook businesses. He wants to be an *architect*."

The derision in his father's tone had made shards of glass whisk through Peter's lungs. Their recent argument over his Oxford curriculum still burned like the stings of a crazed swarm of bees.

"You should let him."

That had been Kenton's reply. Surprise had surged through Peter, quickly followed by joy and relief, the immensity so great that he almost melted into a puddle.

"He's smart and talented. Smarter than both of us and brave enough to forge a new kind of future. Don't rein him in."

Please, please, please, he'd found himself thinking. Every part of him had tensed and he'd risen to his toes. Waited, waited, prayed. He hadn't expected Kenton to be his champion, to intervene, to provide this last chance. But maybe...please...maybe...please...could Kenton sway his father's mind?

"No."

"Oh, John." Kenton's voice was sick with disappointment and despair, the very kind churning in Peter's stomach. His vision had swum. Kenton hadn't been able to budge his best friend's unrelenting stubbornness, but he'd believed in Peter. He'd tried. And Peter had never stopped being grateful.

The memory faded. Peter pushed his blanket aside. He was uncomfortably hot. How strange that, of the memories that flashed through his mind, the one he recalled most clearly was the day Kenton tried to convince his father Peter deserved to be his own man. Gratitude and fondness for Kenton rose and made him want to unequivocally deny any wrongdoing committed by the man, especially a wrongdoing so heinous. Except, his sense of fairness wouldn't quite let him. Instead, something that felt a lot like betrayal demanded he consider the unthinkable.

CHAPTER FOUR

The next morning, after church services, Anne arrived at the surgery determined to put her foolishness about Mr. Matthews behind her. He was a handsome man with an appealing manner, interesting and somewhat mysterious, and he'd prompted a few unexpected, fanciful feelings, but that was it. Yesterday she'd acted like a ninny, which she had no intention of doing again. So she paused with her hand on the doorknob and took two deep breaths. Then, with a silent and stern admonishment to herself, she came through the back door, greeted Mrs. Pettigrew, and hung her hat and wrap on an empty peg.

"He drank his tea and porridge, and now Owen Weaver is having a word," the cook-housekeeper said, stared into the pot she stirred and sighed. "I thought myself past the shock, but seeing young Weaver's empty sleeve today distressed me as much as his first time back at Sunday worship. The poor lad."

Owen wasn't a lad. He was a man, an army veteran who'd sacrificed his arm in service of the Crown. Both he and Anne had grown up in Buttermere and been schoolmates, and when he was sent to the Crimea Anne wrote a few newsy letters to give him a taste of home and to let him know his friends were thinking of him. She'd barely seen Owen since his return, but she'd noticed a change as significant as the loss of his arm—the joviality that had been an integral part of him was gone. He still had the rough look of a Crimean soldier, his beard and hair untrimmed.

"I wonder why he's here," she said, donning a fresh apron.

"Perhaps he brought a message from his father." Mrs. Pettigrew shrugged. "Mr. Carter's gone to Loweswater. He said to tell you Mr. Matthews spent a fitful night but hasn't developed vomiting or fever."

"That's encouraging," Anne said. Edwin had planned to visit several patients in the vicinity of Loweswater as long as Mr. Matthews's condition allowed. She didn't expect him back until afternoon now. Excepting an emergency, the day should be quiet.

She left the kitchen, tapped on the closed convalescent room door and opened it. Mr. Matthews's color appeared somewhat improved, but tension etched his face. She'd seen many people worried, in pain, grieving, and had acquired the ability to recognize even the subtler signs: the tautness of a jaw muscle, deeper facial lines, a compression of the lips.

"Good morning," she said, entering the room.

Owen stood, and both men greeted Anne.

"I should be going," Owen said. "I'll bring my father up to date," he added, directing his words to Mr. Matthews. Then he left.

Anne hurried after and caught him at the surgery front door. "Owen, wait."

He stopped and turned, and the corners of his mouth lifted. It was small as smiles went, but his eyes creased, making the expression one of unquestionable warmth.

Careful not to glance where his arm used to be, Anne looked directly into his eyes. There was a new steadiness there that had been missing since his return from the Crimea, so she proceeded with her questions. "How are you? Have you decided to seek work in London?" He'd mentioned the possibility when they chatted a few minutes after last Sunday's services.

"I'm...feeling more myself," he acknowledged. "My father has set me a few tasks. I'll decide about London once those are accomplished."

Anne nodded. Thank goodness Constable Weaver had found something for his son.

"You'll be shocked to hear our old schoolmaster offered to provide me a reference."

"No!" Anne crimped her lips, trying to restrain her smile. "Mr. Peasley?"

Owen's teeth flashed in a quick smile, and laughter rumbled in his chest as he nodded. A teasing glint sparked his eyes. Here was the schoolmate she remembered from before the war. Anne's breath caught, and she chortled in shared amusement.

"He reminded me of the time I slipped a cricket into his pocket. Remember? Fortune smiled that day. Each time he started to speak, the cricket chirped. He couldn't figure out where the chirping was coming from, and our classmates were in stitches!" Owen rolled his eyes. "He knew I'd done it, because, who else would?"

They both chuckled.

"You must have washed the schoolroom windows and swept that floor more than all the other students combined," Anne teased. "At least during our tenure no other mischief-maker compared."

"Mr. Peasley claims I've never been equaled. Except, now he tells me my cheeky disposition made me a favorite."

Laughing, Anne shook her head in wonder. "It's good to see you, Owen. Take care. If you decide to go to London, be sure and stop by before you leave."

"I'll do that, Anne."

He tipped his hat and exited, on the forecourt greeting Andrew Snow, who was coming in. Tightness cinched Anne's stomach when she saw her suitor. She'd not been face-to-face with him since Thursday when he'd proposed and she'd told him she needed time to think it over.

He entered the waiting area and snatched his hat from his head. Mouth stretched tight, he gave a short nod, avoiding her gaze. "I'm here to speak to Mr. Matthews about his horse."

So, he was still hurt, confused, and angry because she hadn't immediately accepted his offer. How to make it better between them? She'd already apologized and tried to explain, but he hadn't understood. Actually, she wasn't even sure he'd *heard* her explanations. She'd managed the situation all wrong.

"Hello, Andrew," she said. "Please, can we talk? Maybe later today?"

His gaze swung and connected to hers, and it was an Andrew she'd never met. His eyes glittered as if full of slivered glass. She understood the answer before he even spoke a word, and she sucked in a shaky breath. *She'd* caused this wound. That she'd done it with the best intentions didn't matter.

"Not today," he said.

She kept her face unchanged. "This way," she replied.

He followed her into Mr. Matthews's room, and she introduced the two men, explaining Mr. Snow owned Buttermere's livery stableyard.

"Thank you for coming," Matthews said. "I understand Red is with you?"

"He is. He settled right in. You needn't worry."

Mr. Matthews looked at Anne. "Would you fetch my coin purse?"

The day he arrived, they'd cut off his coat. She'd removed the small bag from the pocket and placed it in his saddlebag, which now lay on the floor beside his boots. When she retrieved it for him, he grimaced.

"Hard to manage with one hand," he said. "Would you mind?" With a gesture and a look, he indicated she should give Andrew the money.

"It's eight pence a day," Andrew said. "Six shillings a week if you'd like to include exercise."

"Thinking I could be gone in a few days is probably optimistic, so we'll make it a week—six shillings—for now."

Anne withdrew the coins and offered them. Andrew hesitated until the wait became uncomfortable, then finally extended his hand. Taking care not to look at him or touch his palm, Anne deposited the six coins and stepped back. He fisted the shillings, and his arm dropped to his side.

Embarrassment swamped Anne. She wanted to sink through the

floor, so she set the coin bag on the table, hurried into the treatment room, and began collecting the supplies she'd need to change Mr. Matthews's dressing. She heard the men exchange a few more words, and then Andrew's footsteps. Instead of passing through to the front, though, he stopped and closed the convalescent room door behind him, granting them privacy from Mr. Matthews's ears.

Anne paused in her work but didn't turn around. *Please, don't challenge me*. Not here, not now.

"Anne, I'm sorry…for acting as I did in front of your patient. I didn't think I could bear to touch you. I've felt so angry and hurt and humiliated. I had no idea you don't share my feelings."

She turned. Those final words had sounded like an accusation. The grim steeliness hadn't softened, either, so she nodded and resisted the urge to fix everything, saying, "I'd like another chance to explain."

Andrew bent his head, rubbed the back of his neck, then donned and secured his hat. "I'll let you know," he said. Then he left, boot heels striking loud and fast, shoulders blocking the light as he passed through the doorway.

When he was gone, Anne took a deep breath. The thought of causing him pain each time they encountered one another was repugnant. If she rejected Andrew's proposal, could their friendship be repaired? How long would the awkwardness between them last? Perhaps she'd be happier leaving Buttermere for a larger city? So many times she'd contemplated leaving. Except, how could she abandon her mother? Aside from a few scattered, distant relatives, Emma was Anne's only remaining family.

A not uncommon streak of resentment flashed through her. It wasn't just lost opportunity to seek and perhaps find love that caused her bitterness. They'd lived on the fringes of the community, never fully accepted, while whispers circled like wild, hungry dogs. She loved her mum, but Mum's pride and stubbornness had kept them in Buttermere even after the deaths of Anne's grandparents. For a moment, loss overcame her. Grandfather Albright had died three years ago. Grandmother the year after. Anne's chest still felt hollow whenever she thought of them.

She exhaled then waited until she felt composed enough to return to Mr. Matthews. A full five minutes. She should have waited longer. The instant she saw him, her face heated. She laid her supplies on his bedside table and prayed he wouldn't comment.

"I'm sorry my business matters put you in an uncomfortable situation," he said.

"I'm fine," she assured him.

"Mr. Snow seemed agitated. I know he embarrassed you, but you needn't feel self-conscious."

Quiet and free of censure, Matthews's voice eased her lingering tension, and Anne sank onto the chair and gave herself to explanation. "Normally he isn't one to divulge private matters, but…his emotions are volatile right now. I did something recently that wounded him. Something I may not be able to fix. This was the first time we'd spoken since it happened."

Was she unreasonable and selfish asking Andrew to wait for a decision? The magnitude of his disappointment and hurt had jerked her heart inside-out, but she had to be sure she made the right choice.

"Does he perhaps want to be more than friends?" Mr. Matthews asked.

"You could tell that?" Anne said. There was a look in his eyes that made her think she could pour her heart out and Mr. Matthews would understand everything. How strange. *He* was the one who should feel alone and afraid and in need of reassurance, yet he was offering friendship to her. Her remaining hesitance drained away. "He proposed, and I haven't given him an answer."

"There's someone else?" Mr. Matthews asked, a new roughness to his voice.

"No."

She should stop. This was so confidential, and she barely knew Mr. Matthews. But his attention was comforting and intoxicating. She wanted more. "It's just…I don't love him the way I want to love the man I marry." She pressed her cold palm to her suddenly hot forehead. "I fear I'm being too idealistic. Andrew is a good man and a valued friend. He'd make a fine husband." Except, apart from her tepid romantic feelings for him, she also worried he cared too much about other's opinions. That would be especially hard if he married someone of Anne's peculiar family situation.

"You have every right to want nothing less than a full-hearted love," Mr. Matthews said.

His approval settled her regrets and doubts. This *was* the most important decision of her life. She deserved to take all the time she needed.

But… She paused. How could the validation of this man—a man who didn't know her—make such a difference? Perhaps because of his sincerity and certainty. And because he'd endured great loss, himself. Did she dare ask about it?

"Were you in love with your fiancée?" she found herself saying.

He blinked. Frowned. Was he going to ignore her? Such a personal question. One she shouldn't have asked.

"I'm sorry, I sh—"

"Louisa was beautiful, and talented, and grace personified. Yes, I loved her." His mouth tightened before he cleared his throat. "She made my life complete."

Anne fought back a brief moment of jealousy, one she didn't want to think about. Matthews had known and lost the kind of love she yearned for. "How long has it been?"

"Three years. We were traveling with my parents. A storm came up. A deluge. We should have stopped, but we were so close to our destination. The river became a torrent. Later I learned it undercut the banks. We were on the bridge when it collapsed. Our carriage went into the water."

Anne gasped. Mr. Matthews glanced at the ceiling and then went on.

"I nearly drowned trying to save them, but it was hopeless from the beginning." His eyes closed for a moment. When they opened, they glimmered wetly, and he fixed his gaze on the ceiling for good.

Anne grasped his hand, and he held on. She was surprised by that.

"At least my betrothal and plans for the future made my parents happy before they died. For the first time in my life, my father was unreservedly pleased and proud." Mr. Matthews released her hand and wiped his eyes, sighed, and rubbed his hand against the blanket atop his chest before clasping Anne's hand again. He flushed. "I'm sorry you're having to put up with me. I'm not myself. Normally I speak of the accident without turning into a watering pot."

She gave his hand a squeeze and made her voice light. "I think, as excuses go, getting shot is a pretty good reason for being discomposed."

He looked at her. "Are you worried you won't find that special person?"

"Yes," she said. If she married Andrew, she thought they would be…content. That wasn't what she'd always wanted, but perhaps it was worse to be like Mr. Matthews, who'd found and lost love before it could be fully realized.

"What about you?" she asked. "I mean, now that…now that Louisa is gone."

"She seemed perfect in every way and was the only one who ever held my interest."

"You don't want to settle," Anne said. Neither did she, yet she hadn't told Andrew no. Would marrying a beloved friend be "settling"? Was it reasonable to expect or desire a true love match in this world? Again, she felt a moment of jealousy at the way Mr. Matthews spoke of his departed fiancée.

"I want children, though," he went on, "so I'll either have to make do or accept a lonely future."

Anne half shivered. What if she refused Andrew and never found the kind of love she dreamed of? Some were eager to marry simply for the joy of children and companionship and security. Wouldn't she be foolish to reject Andrew? And perhaps, once married, after she and he had experienced that most intimate sharing of themselves, true love would burst from its chrysalis and fly.

"My cousin assures me there's room in my heart for someone else," Mr. Matthews continued. He sounded uncertain, as if he didn't quite believe it. "But he has always been the optimistic sort."

Anne gave a nod. "I agree with your cousin. I think our hearts have an infinite capacity for love. I didn't know your Louisa, but I imagine she'd want you to find happiness. I certainly would." He released her hand and rubbed his forehead, and Anne stood, suddenly embarrassed by her admission. "I've kept you talking too long. Did Mr. Carter give you a dose of pain tonic before he left?"

"No, and I could use one."

"Let me get it, and then you can rest awhile. We'll change your dressing later."

He remained quiet and she left.

In the treatment room she measured a dose of laudanum into a small cup of water, and a soft warmth filled her chest. She and Mr. Matthews had exchanged private, poignant details about themselves, and they'd forged a bond that felt uncommonly strong between patient and caregiver. How sad that it would end when he recovered and left Buttermere—which was what would unquestionably happen.

She returned to Mr. Matthews, and he drank the laudanum down without a grimace. They exchanged a smile as he passed her the empty cup, and their fingers brushed, and yearning blossomed in Anne's chest, breasts, and pelvis. For that reason, she said something about his resting and fled to the treatment room with a need to choke down one inescapable truth:

His single touch aroused more desire than Andrew's most fervent kiss.

CHAPTER FIVE

The next day, the sounds outside Peter's room kept him entertained. The treatment room, where Carter examined and tended to patients, was directly across the hall. Even with the door closed, he heard most of what occurred. The surgeon was having a busy day, even with Anne helping.

As long as Peter lay still, his shoulder and back pain were tolerable; the whirling sensation and subsequent nausea happened when he turned his head. The headache was constant, but the axe didn't split his brain unless he moved or coughed or laughed. Or got angry. So he lay still, listened to the birds in the tree outside the open window, or the work going on in the other room, and tried not to plague himself with the constant worry of who had been trying to kill him.

The conversations of Carter and Anne and their patients were welcome distractions: A boy with an earache, trying hard to be brave and not cry. Another boy, a tree climber, who fell. He whimpered, then yelped and cried when Carter straightened the broken bones in his arm. Then Anne held the arm of the boy—Elmer—and talked to him while Carter splinted it. Peter commiserated with the lad. He sounded about twelve, and Peter had done the exact same thing and broken the same arm at that age. His mother had cried and his father had laughed and said he hoped Peter would use better judgment in the future. Remembering made Peter's heart pinch. He missed them.

Next came a man from the nearby Dale Head Slate Mine who'd injured his leg. A woman with a festering burn. A grandmother with a cough. As Peter listened, his admiration for Carter grew. The man was patient, conscientious, and confident in his knowledge. He treated each person with kindness and courtesy. As for Anne, she possessed more patience and compassion than anyone he'd ever met.

Carter maintained proper interactions with her, Peter noticed, but the man's tone of voice changed whenever he spoke to Anne. Became warm, relaxed, and held a true and well-worn familiarity. There was a good deal of silence between the pair, too, as if they were so accustomed to one another and working together that they didn't require instructions or explanations.

Somewhere in the house a clock chimed noon. Carter stuck his head in Peter's door.

"Feeling better?"

"Entertained," Peter said, pointing toward the treatment room on the other side of the hall. "When I wasn't cringing."

Carter cocked his head, and they both listened to the voices of Anne and Mrs. Pettigrew, which carried from the kitchen. Carter nodded as if he understood. "I'm making patient visits this afternoon. Anne will be here. Take some laudanum after you eat and try to sleep for a while."

"I've discovered the sounds of the breeze, birds, and bees are downright soporific. I—" Peter broke off, suddenly realizing Carter had used Anne's given name again. He'd called her Miss Albright all morning while they tended their patients, but in front of Peter he didn't make much effort to address her properly. Then, like a key in a lock, understanding turned and clicked in Peter's mind. Using her given name in front of him was deliberate, meant to apprise him that the surgeon and nurse didn't share a simple congenial working association but a close and personal bond. Anne had denied anything more intimate than friendship, but apparently Carter disagreed.

Peter gritted his teeth, and pain pulsed in his head, going from the tapping of a woodpecker to the solid whack of an axe. Then he relaxed his jaw. He didn't have the right to feel perturbed. He certainly shouldn't feel protective of Anne and at odds with Carter!

Yet...he did.

Yesterday, he and Anne had told one another of experiences that had affected them deeply. He felt a continued connection with her now, one far stronger than two days of acquaintance warranted. What was going on here? Had his brush with death made him vulnerable and needy? Perhaps, he acknowledged, but it hadn't made him imagine qualities in Anne that didn't exist. She was a unique and wonderful woman. No one listening while she performed her work duties today could doubt how special she was. So he couldn't blame Carter for acting proprietary.

But, couldn't *he* act proprietary as well? Damn it. Why *not* let the good surgeon know that, as much as Peter admired his doctoring skill, he found Carter's manners unbecoming in a man of his position? Unless the two were set to wed, Carter should be calling his assistant Miss Albright in the presence of company.

"I'm grateful for the fine care you and Miss Albright have given me," Peter began. Then: "At first I thought her your wife or fiancée, the way you refer to her as Anne."

Carter folded his arms and tipped his chin, clearly unmoved by the rebuke. "You were a stranger who came to us by way of violence. She's a lovely woman, and unmarried. You're often alone together. I have a brotherly affection for her, and want you to know she...doesn't lack protection."

Peter gave a nod, wondering if that was the whole truth. When Anne had spoken of her dilemma regarding Snow, she hadn't mentioned Carter. Did she truly not see him as a potential suitor?

"I'm glad you keep watch," he finally said. "She deserves it."

Carter gave a nod. His arms dropped, and he turned to leave.

"Hold up. I owe you for the operation and the care I've received."

The surgeon paused. "There's no need to settle your account now."

"That's kind of you," Peter said, "but I want you to know there's enough in my money bag to cover your fee should I take a turn for the worse, and I expect you to take what's owed."

"Very well," Carter said. Then he left.

Not long after, Anne brought soup. She propped up Peter's head, sat beside him, and fed him a spoonful: chicken with thick, tasty broth and noodles. He closed his eyes and enjoyed the comfort that spread clear through to his bones with the first swallow.

"Mrs. Pettigrew cut the noodles up very small to make it easier for you to eat."

"Mmm. I'm beginning to understand Mrs. Pettigrew is a pearl among women. And she"—he laughed, remembering his surprise at hearing them—"sings the most delightful sea shanties. Is there a Mr. Pettigrew?"

"She's a widow, but she's a mite older than you. Perhaps you've an uncle looking for a wife?"

Peter stared at Anne, taken aback. She was teasing him. He liked the glint in her eyes, and that sassy smile, so he responded in kind. "Perhaps the quality of her cooking overcomes the difference in our ages."

"A few compliments like that and she'll be cooking all your favorites all the time."

"Truly?" Peter said. "Because I'm very fond of treacly spice cake."

Anne grinned. "I'll tell her."

That smile filled Peter with a sense of satisfaction not unlike the feeling left behind after a good belly laugh. He *was* feeling better, because today he saw little things he hadn't noticed yesterday, such as a scatter of freckles that sprinkled Anne's nose like nutmeg afloat a creamy eggnog.

He swallowed another mouthful of the fine noodle soup.

"I'm happy you feel well enough to request something that pleases you," Anne said, her eyebrows raised. "Perhaps you'd be able to dictate letters? You still need to inform your employer what happened."

Peter had an answer ready. "The rector offered to help with my correspondence. He assured me it wouldn't be a burden."

Anne nodded, her concerns seemingly mollified, then offered another spoonful of soup. And then another.

"Once you feel well enough to become bored, we could have a game of backgammon," she suggested. "Although, I'll understand if you refuse. Losing is never fun." She gave him a look at once both innocent and teasing.

"I've found an expert, have I? Would you take unfair advantage of a man at his lowest?"

"Certainly not. You'll be nicely distracted and enjoy yourself immensely."

"How kind of you to suggest a diversion for my mind."

"My pleasure," Anne said.

Their gazes met and held for a long moment, and they fell quiet. Peace settled over Peter and he realized that for this short time he'd forgotten his pain.

"I overheard you working today, and it provided a welcome distraction," Peter said. "Buttermere residents must be very grateful, to have a nurse of your caliber living here. And Carter. He's a fine surgeon. Buttermere is lucky to have him, too. You said as much when I arrived, but..."

"Very lucky," Anne agreed. "I'm especially fortunate. He treats me like a respected colleague. Some physicians and surgeons still regard nurses as either disreputable or on a par with the lowliest servant."

Peter's forehead creased. "Surely Florence Nightingale's work has changed such antiquated notions. Queen Victoria and Prince Albert have made no secret of their admiration."

"Too many physicians regard Miss Nightingale as an exception," Anne said. "But not Mr. Carter. Attitudes are changing. Attitudes about all sorts of things. Just...slower than women like myself would like."

The space between her eyebrows creased, and for a moment that frown puzzled Peter, but then he realized: The scandal of her parentage. He'd forgotten it in his contemplation of her beauty and kind competence.

"I love being a nurse," she went on. "It feeds my heart."

She'd neatly turned the conversation away from her difficulties, but he let her.

"How is that?"

"I like helping people. Sometimes I'm present during the largest crisis of someone's life, and I'm the anchor people hold on to. If my being there makes things even a little more bearable, then I'm happy."

"But that's not every day," Peter pointed out.

"You'd be surprised how rewarding it is providing even small services. Like...helping someone eat soup."

Peter started to chuckle, but he stopped when it made both his head and back wound pulse. "Don't make me laugh," he begged. "It hurts."

"I'll restrain myself," she agreed, and offered another spoonful of soup with more information about herself. "I find disease and everything associated with a medical practice fascinating. Mr. Carter enjoys teaching, and I've learned a lot from him."

What a different woman this was from Louisa, Peter found himself thinking. What would his fiancée have thought of her? Sadly, both she and his mother would have likely found Anne peculiar. Or maybe "eccentric," if they'd been inclined toward kindness. They certainly wouldn't have gone as far as "admirable."

The realization made him uncomfortable. His mother had praised Louisa, a woman much like herself. How often had she commented that Louisa would make her son the perfect viscountess? And, Louisa had assured him she'd devote herself to entertaining his political and business associates in order to strengthen Peter's affiliations and influence. He could hardly imagine Anne finding much joy in that, in subordinating her intelligence to pursuit of his goals and those of his estate; in chatting with the wives of his colleagues, women who'd been coddled all their lives and whose primary concerns were social ones. Especially not when the reward—such as having a part in the passage of some much-needed law—came far too infrequently.

"I envy your satisfaction," Peter said.

"You don't enjoy your work?"

"It's agreeable, but I do it because I must, not because I love it." He gave a shrug. "I shouldn't complain. Most men do whatever they must to support themselves and their family. It's a fortunate person who loves his work."

Anne stared at him. Her smile was warm, but her amber eyes held a question.

"I wanted to design things," he answered. "Bridges and buildings. Big things, like the Crystal Palace. What a challenge *that* would be."

The center of Peter's chest got warm—no, hot. He'd never confessed this to even Louisa. If he had, she wouldn't have understood. He'd wanted to be an engineer or an architect. He'd been told he had a gift for math and design, and he'd spent hours studying and sketching. For a time he'd denied that the demands of his ancestral duties would dominate his life, while again and again his parents insisted family and title came first. Building things, they'd said, wasn't even a suitable hobby. A long line of Viscount Easterbrooks had cared for all that would someday belong to Peter; he owed it to his present, past, and future family to be an exemplary custodian. His time, attention, and efforts were to be directed to Easterbrook affairs and nothing else. When he wasn't at school, he was to be at his father's side, learning to step into his shoes.

His father.

Both he and Peter's grandfather had always stressed good stewardship, but Peter's father worried Peter's fascination with engineering and science—and Peter's desire to incorporate them into managing the Easterbrook holdings—would be disastrous. Peter had seen it as the only way to keep up with the changing world. His father had thought he was "following a passing fashion, this fixation on scientific method," and had urged Peter to be even more careful and conservative than he himself had been while watching the Easterbrook estate decline over the years. It was a major bone of contention between them, and one of their last arguments had concerned the aging bridge that—unbeknownst to them all—would destroy Peter's family and change his life. Peter had wanted the bridge rebuilt using modern technology, and reasoned it would serve them far better and longer despite the cost. His father had believed a simple repair would work just as well. Tired of the arguing, of the dire warnings that under Peter's stewardship all the Easterbrook assets would be lost, Peter had let the issue drop.

His fault.

He should have pressed harder, longer, not given up. He'd never do so again. Not when he knew another way was better and he had the means to effect the correction. Now, whether he was buying a business or giving a tenant a new roof, Peter's goal was to always move things forward. It wasn't just about maintaining or managing, but about making things better, about making things *safe*.

That was what made the financial risks worthwhile. That was what was going on with the mine up north.

The clink of a spoon against china drew his attention back to Anne, and she gave a slow nod. "Well, if they can, a person should always do what they love." She paused, blinked, and added, "Doing so can be as profoundly affecting as the contents of Mr. Carter's medicine cupboard. So, if it'll comfort you, I'll bring pencils and ruler and a sketchpad. You'll eventually be able to slip your arm out of the sling and move your hand and wrist. You may not draw up plans for the next Osborne House right away, but perhaps that'll come in time. Maybe *next* week," she offered with a smile. "You have to do what you love."

Peter's heart flipped. Anne made it sound so simple: As if not designing buildings was denying an integral part of himself. As if filling that empty space would help him heal both physically and mentally. He *was* always scribbling and sketching, but designing? After all this time, he didn't know if he could.

What would he design? *Something.*

"Thank you," he said.

A youth appeared in the doorway. "Miss Albright? Is there anything I can do for you?"

She glanced over at him, looking surprised. "Oh. Come in, Michael, and meet Mr. Matthews." As the boy advanced to Anne's side she added, "This is Michael Elmore. He helps out here after school and on weekends."

"You're the man the poacher shot," Michael said, staring at Peter. "Everyone's talking about it."

Peter supposed the whole village knew of the incident, and were curious. "I'm afraid so."

"If you need anything from the mercantile, sir, let me know and I'll fetch it," Michael said, looking eager to please. That made Peter smile through a sudden wave of fatigue.

"Thank you. I'll remember."

The boy excused himself when he said nothing further. After a moment, Peter looked at Anne, loath to say so, but it couldn't be put off.

"I think I'm ready to rest now."

She nodded, rose, and carried out his dishes.

Peter adjusted his pillow, exhausted though his mind whirled with thoughts of architecture, of thoughts of his abandoned past. Anne had really hit upon something. How had she understood what he himself hadn't? Architecture wasn't only something he loved. It was *part* of him. Even today, he analyzed every building he saw. His fingers itched with a sudden desire to grip a pencil, a desire as strong as the determination he felt whenever he started up a new mountain: his other passion. He'd begun mountaineering when he stopped taking classes intended for a budding architect, and each year those mountains had gotten higher and the ascents more demanding. He'd felt freest on those mountainsides where most men didn't venture. Unfettered.

His parents hadn't liked it, his sudden love of mountaineering, but they'd said at least it was a pursuit of gentlemen and only took him away once or twice a year, rather than devouring all his waking attention. He'd frequently taken Arthur with him, and they had grudgingly accepted his hobby in spite of its danger, perhaps because they understood that when he stood atop a summit his soul opened wide.

Just like when he saw a beautiful building or an amazing bridge and considered what it had taken to create.

Very much like when he'd first looked into Anne's honey-gold eyes.

CHAPTER SIX

It was late that afternoon when the jangle of the front door bell woke Peter. A man's footsteps approached, accompanied by the rustle of skirts and lighter tread of a woman, and a welcoming grin was already on Peter's face when Arthur and Belinda filled the doorway, Belinda holding their six-month-old daughter.

He barely had time to acknowledge them before a small boy squeezed out from between the couple. Belinda started to call her son back, but Peter held up a staying hand. "It's all right," he said. "I'd hoped he'd remember me enough from Rebecca's christening to not be leery. Come in, and welcome."

Mimicking a horse, three-year-old Henry galloped around the room, stopped at Peter's bedside, and whinnied.

"What a fine stallion," Peter said. "Would you like a carrot?"

Henry gave a few horse-like bobs of his head and pawed his pretend-hoof against the floor. Peter withdrew an invisible carrot from beneath his covers and offered it, flat-palmed. Horse-like, the boy took the carrot in his mouth, chewed, whinnied, and galloped to the window.

Belinda moved close, bent and offered her cheek. Rebecca,

securely held in her mother's arms, gave an excited squeal as she tipped, and Peter kissed the curve of his cousin's wife's cheek and inhaled Belinda's lavender and Rebecca's own scent, which was a combination of her mother and something else he couldn't quite identify.

Belinda sat in a chair and settled Rebecca on her lap. Arthur closed the door and dragged a second seat to Peter's bedside.

"She's beautiful," Peter said. The infant was healthy looking, her rosy-cheeked face and brown curls framed by a charming, lace-trimmed pink bonnet. "I see she's putting my teething ring to good use."

"She loves shaking it," Belinda said, gazing down at her daughter, who clutched the ivory ring that was one of several gifts Peter had sent. A silver cat charm and two tiny bells dangled from the hoop.

"We won't stay long. The children get restless," Arthur spoke up. "Here, son," he called, and Henry came to his side. From his pocket Arthur withdrew a wooden horse and a figure of a man and handed them to the boy. Henry dropped to the rug then reached up toward his father, who fished in his pocket a second time, removed something and held it up for Peter to see: a miniature saddle fashioned of wool, complete with tiny stirrups.

"Belinda made it," Arthur said. He passed it to Henry, who began playing with his three toys.

"I'm glad you came and brought the children. They've grown so much!"

Peter hoped his voice and reactions seemed natural. Getting a good look at Belinda had unsettled him. While his cousin's wife watched her child, he stabbed a questioning look Arthur's way, and his cousin answered with a grim stare. Arthur had said Belinda had lost weight, but Peter hadn't imagined *this*. She was gaunt, her cheeks hollow. Except for a feverish-looking flush on the crest of each cheekbone, she looked colorless and tired, and while her lips curved into smiles, her eyes didn't.

"It's horrible, you being in these circumstances," she said, glancing at Peter. "I was shocked." Steadying her drooling infant, she gave a bounce with her knee. "How is your wound? Are you in pain?"

"My head hurts more than my back. When it's necessary, I take a pain tonic. It keeps the worst at bay."

Belinda nodded, stood, and began walking back and forth, patting Rebecca's back as if she needed comforting, and jouncing her a bit.

"How have you been, Belinda?" Peter asked. "Has it been difficult to meet your community responsibilities now that you have two children?"

"I've been well," the woman replied, if a bit stiffly. "And childrearing is no more difficult for me than it is for any other woman. At any rate, Buttermere's population is small, and Arthur's congregation doesn't require much of me."

"Ah," Peter said. He couldn't help remembering that, shortly after their marriage, Arthur had confided his wife's transition from aristocrat to rector's wife was difficult. The parish had known Belinda as Kenton's daughter and deferred to her for years, and then suddenly she was expected to assist them in times of sickness and hardship. The locals had felt uncomfortable placing her in the position of friend and helper, and, according to Arthur, they'd never quite stopped regarding her as an interloper. But he'd said she kept trying. "How are your parents?"

Belinda stopped at the window. "They're healthy and busy with their own concerns. The village recently honored Father for his beneficence: the foundation he started several years ago to assist any slate miner's family whose man is injured, disabled, or killed, and the Buttermere School, which he built and continues to support."

The reminder of Viscount Kenton's constant philanthropy raised a question in Peter's mind. Was it possible for a man so altruistic to be a rapist? *Of course,* said common sense. Couldn't guilt, or the desire to affect public opinion, be the cause of a wealthy man's gifts? And yet, Peter didn't want to believe. For the past two days, thoughts of what Arthur had disclosed stayed close at hand. Anne's very existence meant *something* had happened, and even after all these years there remained people who believed the something had been rape. Peter's sense of fairness demanded he consider the possibility, even as doing so made him feel a traitor. He wanted to meet Emma Albright and smash his sliver of doubt into smithereens.

There was a tap at the door, which opened. Anne appeared, and her smile wilted as her eyes widened.

"Excuse me. I didn't realize who was here. I mean, I heard voices, and thought you might want refreshment."

Peter glanced at Belinda, who whirled, putting her back to the window. "You may serve tea. My son will have lemonade."

That pompous tone. It might have been an Egyptian queen to a house slave, and embarrassment flooded Peter as Anne's mouth pinched into a thin line and she closed the door.

One corner of Arthur's mouth grew tight enough to crease his cheek.

"Don't look at me that way," Belinda commanded.

"I've never heard you use that tone," Arthur said. "Not to anyone."

Belinda's mouth flattened, her hip cocked, and her toe tapped. "I'm sorry my tone wasn't sister-sweet," she said. Then, for the first time since their arrival, she gazed straight at Peter. "This is one of the few things Arthur and I argue about. He thinks Miss Albright and I should be bosom friends."

"You should at least be cordial," Arthur corrected.

The shock that had frozen Peter melted away. His tongue released and he said, "I'm sorry I placed you in an uncomfortable position. I didn't think of anything but the pleasure of seeing you and the children again." Honestly, though, he felt worse for Anne. Was it always like this between the two women? He supposed it was.

"It's no matter," Belinda said. She returned to her chair and settled the baby on her lap. "Our duties sometimes require us to work in concert."

"Oh?" Peter asked. "When is that?"

"Any crisis—death, injury, or sickness—that requires Miss Albright's presence. I'm expected to be of service in those same situations. It helps that she's usually tending the ailing person, while I'm looking after the family." Belinda leaned back against the chair and her shoulders sagged.

"Do you have to work with her mother, too?"

"Not often," Arthur said.

"Thank God," Belinda added sotto voce.

"Belinda!"

"I've done a lot for you, Arthur," his wife said. "More than you'll ever know," she went on, then stopped and breathed. "I don't regret any of it," she added in a milder tone. "I want you to be happy and proud of me. But I draw the line at making Miss Albright and her mother part of my family."

"I've never asked you to associate with Emma Albright," Arthur replied, "but Miss Albright is likely Rebecca and Henry's aunt. That in itself demands courtesy."

Belinda gazed at her daughter and shook her head.

Arthur rubbed his earlobe then looked out the window. "I'm sorry, Peter. We haven't all been together in months, and now we've subjected you to our worst doings."

"I still think you have a perfect marriage," Peter said. "Everyone has difficult moments."

Arthur gave a strained-sounding chuckle. "Yes, well... Your opinion might change if you were around us more often."

Belinda's head came up. "Arthur!"

She sounded hurt, and she looked like a rejected puppy.

The door opened. Mrs. Pettigrew entered, bearing a tray laden with teapot, cups and saucers, and a small glass of what appeared to be lemonade. The appearance of the cook instead of Anne eased Peter's tension.

"I've biscuits, ma'am, if the young gentleman may have one?"

Henry scrambled to his feet and ran jabbering to his mother. Peter thought he made out the word "Please?"

Belinda smiled and stroked a lock of hair from her son's forehead, and for the first time since they'd arrived Peter saw the Belinda he knew. Or at least the ghost of her.

"Yes, dear. Sit down and let me help you."

Henry sat on the rug, bent and crossed his legs.

"I'll take his lemonade, if you'd be so kind, Mrs. Pettigrew," Belinda went on. The condescending tone she'd used with Anne had vanished, and she was all kindness and light. Silence fell, and Peter watched young Henry enjoying his afternoon treat. When the boy offered a nibble of his biscuit to his toy horse, Peter met Arthur's gaze and they wordlessly shared their amusement. Yet, as much as it warmed Peter's heart seeing his cousin in the role of doting parent, it made another part of Peter's chest ache with emptiness. His and Louisa's children might have looked much like Arthur's.

Unexpectedly, his mind suddenly leapt to Anne. She'd make a wonderful mother: loving and kind yet firm.

Belinda stood, set down her empty cup, and flashed a smile to rival a circus performer's. "We should get the children home," she said.

"Oh," said Peter, disappointed. His mug remained half-full, its heat still warming his hand. His cousin hesitated, then set down his unfinished tea and rose. With commendable efficiency, his wife orchestrated their goodbyes and ushered her family out the door, Arthur leaving last and giving Peter a look of resigned solidarity.

A few minutes later, Ann swept in and began collecting dishware.

Peter raised his mug to show he hadn't finished. "I'll keep mine, if I may?"

Anne paused, then set the tray she carried atop the chest of drawers, her creamy complexion flushed red. "I'm embarrassed you saw me spoken to in such a way."

"There's no need to feel self-conscious," Peter reassured her. "If anyone should be embarrassed, it is Mrs. Jennett." He paused. "I know the way she spoke to you distressed her husband. He scolded her."

Anne's eyes widened, and she grew taller and straighter. "In other circumstances I would have taken her to task for acting so high and mighty, but with you, Mr. Jennett, and her children here, I thought it best not to aggravate the situation."

Peter gave a nod. "Probably wise."

"We..." Anne added Henry's glass to the waiting tray and picked it up. "...have a history, Mrs. Jennett and I."

"You must find it difficult to be around her then," Peter offered. "I'm sorry you were uncomfortable."

"Usually she ignores me, and I ignore her," the nurse said with a frown. "I'm not sure that's for the best, but it's easy."

Peter wanted to say something. Before he could figure out what, however, Anne had shrugged and was gone.

CHAPTER SEVEN

The day after the rector and her half-sister's visit, Anne looked into the sick room and found Mr. Matthews standing at the window. The rose-strewn bedcover hung from his bare shoulders, his dark hair bristled in fifty different directions, and the way he'd propped himself against the frame poked her nurse's intuition. He was pale and breathing fast and deep.

"You might have tried sitting up before you tried walking," Anne chided. How had he even gotten out of bed on his own? His head had to be spinning, pounding, or both.

She went to his left. When he straightened, she slipped her arm about his waist, atop the knitted blanket, and tucked herself next to him. His arm came around her shoulders, and he leaned against her. As he did, heat flared down her side.

"Do you have a fever?" She pressed her palm to the side of his face, which was warm. Maybe warmer than it should be. Bristly facial hair prickled her skin, and similar heat spread from her palm to her neck and face. "You're going to have a beard in a few more days."

"It only took my getting shot to make me fashionable," he quipped. "No one will know me."

She knew he felt terrible. What made the silly man stand there and joke?

"Let's get you back to bed."

She urged him away from the window, but he locked his knees. His hand went to the window rail and he said, "How about the chair."

Those words might have asked permission, but his tone didn't. Still, the stubborn fool swayed like laundry in a breeze.

"If you go down, I'll end up going down with you and I'd rather not." She put more strength into her pull, pointing out, "I need to change your dressing." She'd take a look at his wound and listen to his lungs, too. If a fever was brewing, it would be due to pneumonia or wound infection.

He released the window rail and turned toward the bed, but when they got to the chair he planted his feet.

"Oh, very well," she muttered. "Have it your way."

She steadied him as he sat. He opened his mouth and took deep breaths.

Anne crossed her arms. "I'll ask Mr. Carter if he has a cushioned chair he could move in here. I don't mind you being up for short periods of time, but I don't want you doing it alone and fainting."

He considered her. "How long will I be here? A long time still, do you think?"

"Well, at the very least I suggest you stay until your head returns to normal, however long that takes."

Peter Matthews's eyes closed. Long inky lashes rested on his cheeks, and somehow they weren't at odds with the masculinity of his face. For a moment Anne sensed how vulnerable he must feel, and how that must contribute to his question. After such a disturbing event as being shot, to have no one but strangers around him...?

She squeezed his arm. "We'll do our best for you." His eyes opened, and she dropped her hand.

"When she brought my morning coffee in, Mrs. Pettigrew said you delivered a baby last night."

"Yes," Anne said, surprised. "My mother had been called away to another patient, so I attended Mrs. Pickford." She thought back. "Mother and daughter are doing well. The Pickfords planned to name any girl Amelia, but the baby was born with a thick fuzz of blonde hair and looks like a little angel with a golden halo. They decided to name her Seraphim."

She was rambling. This man was too handsome. She dragged her gaze from his blue eyes, tugged the blanket from his shoulders and let it fall to his hips. Picking up its ends, she wrapped them around his waist, engulfing his drawers-clad hips and legs, leaving his chest bare except for the narrow bandage that also looped over his shoulder.

"Why aren't you wearing your sling?" she asked.

Moving behind him, she unknotted his bandage. As she began rolling it up, he raised his arms away from his sides and winced.

"I took it off. In case I needed my hand to steady myself."

"Ah." Twisting the fabric of his bandage around his chest, using first one hand and then the other, Anne leaned close, her face near the angle of Peter Matthews's neck. He smelled of the soap she'd used to wash him. Her fingers, brushing against his warm skin, tingled. The muscular planes of his back rose and fell with his breathing, and warmth assailed her as if her whole body blushed. It was so, so wrong to be overcome by this unwanted attraction and to have such feelings. No other patient had ever affected her this way.

She clamped her teeth together, feeling less like a nurse with every passing moment and more like a simple woman. These ever stronger romantic feelings made her twitch with shame. Nursing was special work, and it required things that no other profession asked of respectable females. In the past two years nursing had received a big boost of respectability and social acceptance because of the accomplishments of Florence Nightingale, so it was crucial Anne maintain an impeccable reputation. For her to discredit herself or her peers would be unforgivable.

How quick people were to believe the worst. Living in Buttermere, she was constantly reminded.

"How does it look?" Mr. Matthews asked. The last of his bandage had fallen away, and with it the dressing. Closed by silk ligatures, the wound had a puckered appearance that it would retain after healing.

"There's a small amount of blood-tinged yellow drainage on the dressing, but not much," she reported. She'd have preferred to see *no* discharge, but this amount wasn't alarming. "There's a little redness around the wound, too, and bruising over your scapula, but that's not unusual."

Anne washed the area, applied ointment and a clean dressing then rolled the bandage back around Mr. Matthews to hold it all in place. Once she had the bandage knotted, she stepped back and admired the snug neatness of it.

"Take some deep breaths while I listen to your chest," she directed.

Matthews complied, and Anne used Edwin's wooden stethoscope baton to listen first to one side of his back and then the other. Air whooshed in and out of his lungs. No wheezing or rubbing or crackling noises.

"Your lungs sound healthy." She straightened and moved around to face him. "So no pneumonia. Your body feels warmer than normal, but that's not unusual after such an injury. It's all encouraging, but you still need rest. Are you ready to go back to bed?"

"I suppose I'd better." He sighed. "Moving around makes everything worse, but lying here all day makes me feel helpless, useless, and restless. This morning I couldn't take it any longer."

"If being out of bed made the pain worse I can give you some laudanum," Anne suggested.

"That makes me feel groggy," Matthews complained. "I'd rather do without unless the pain becomes too bad to ignore."

"Take it at night at least. You'll sleep better," she explained. Then she spared a moment to consider his predicament. She'd been too busy to see him most of yesterday, and Edwin had been making house calls, so being alone had probably left him feeling lost. Had the rector helped him contact his employer and write any other letters he needed to send off?

"I'm sorry I haven't brought the sketchpad yet," she said. "I thought there was one at home, but I couldn't find it. I'll buy one from Danvers Retail. I could find a novel for you, although reading—like anything needing great focus—might prove difficult right now. I can also bring Mr. Carter's chess set in. You might find a game with

Reverend Jennett or Mr. Carter. Or there are cards. We could play patience. Or backgammon," she added with a smirk. "Yes, we should probably play backgammon."

"You have no shame, challenging a sick man?"

She couldn't hold the bark of laughter in. "You'll have to wait and see."

"Are you suggesting we make a wager? What would be the stakes?"

His sudden grin made Anne's stomach squeeze. Appalled, she clamped a hand to her middle and reminded herself of all her previous admonitions. What was she doing? Teasing? Joking? *Flirting*?

She ducked away and straightened the bed, and luck was with her as he stood and returned to the mattress with no more assistance than simply taking her hand to steady himself. He swallowed hard and moaned a little as he laid back, though, so she knew his head was still a source of misery and instructed him to lie on his side. Once he'd found a comfortable position, she tucked the blanket around him.

He turned to look at her. Pale and surely tired, perhaps he would rest if she left him. She should prepare for the afternoon surgery patients soon anyway, but...just a few more minutes. She didn't want to leave.

She straightened and caught sight of gossamer filaments stretching across a corner of the ceiling over the bed. Ah. *That* was how she could—innocently—extend their time together.

"A spider web!" she said. "Mrs. Pettigrew would have a fit and be horribly embarrassed she missed it. I'll get the broom, and it'll be our little secret."

"Please don't," Matthews said, surprising her.

"Why ever not? I promise not to drop the spider on your head."

"Well..." He hesitated. "I've been watching her spin, and she's kept me entertained while I lie here. I can't help feeling a little proud of her accomplishment."

"Leave it? Are you sure?" Anne asked. She wouldn't like lying under a spider, but she supposed, if it gave Mr. Matthews some small degree of entertainment, it wouldn't hurt to leave the daddy-longlegs undisturbed.

"Positive. And now you understand how bored I am when you're not here."

"All right," she said, blushing and hoping he wouldn't notice. Perhaps, in addition to relieving his tedium and filling time when she couldn't be with him, the spider would serve as a distraction from pain. "But you mustn't overdo it again, getting up on your own and then standing at the window. Promise me. Have one of us help you. I don't want to pick you up off the floor."

Mr. Matthews gave a nod.

"I suppose I can't begrudge you your time away," he said after a moment. "Helping new life into the world the way you did last night must be extra special."

Anne settled on the chair he had vacated and smiled in reminiscence. "The first baby I delivered on my own was Robin Blythe. He's ten years old now. Every time I see Robin, I grin. I can't help myself."

"I can quite understand," Mr. Matthews said. "But after our talk the other day I thought about those crises you mentioned, the ones where you feel you can *really help people*. Those must be difficult for you. I can tell you really care, and for something to go wrong..."

He'd thought further about that conversation? Anne was both flattered and flustered. "Yes." She hesitated, thinking of the patients she'd cared for and their families. "It's hard to see people through bad times, and even through the ends of their lives, but it's also an honor."

She couldn't seem to look away from Mr. Matthews's face, his slightly curved mouth and warm, approving gaze. And then he said, "I hope this community realizes how fortunate they are to have a nurse with your skill—and better yet, your heart."

Anne blushed into her very core. This compliment wasn't just about what she did, but about who she was.

Her heart expanded until it filled her chest. Edwin would thank her and tell her when she did a medical procedure well, but otherwise she received little praise from him—and never about sensitivity to her patients. Most of the villagers appreciated her, she knew. Sometimes, when they ushered her into their homes or she met them as they came through the door of the surgery, their faces filled with relief. They trusted both her mother's and her nursing judgments, yet both Anne and Emma were set apart from other Buttermere residents; the taint of the old scandal had never left them. How many summer Sundays had the Kenton family's cold-eyed stares filled the pit of Anne's stomach with ice while, like an orchestra following a conductor, the congregation's gazes swayed to her pew? Gossip always intensified on those summer days the Kentons resided at Pennyton Park. It made her imagine how much easier it would be to care for people who didn't know everything about her, and who hadn't judged her mother. And yet, she couldn't stop caring about them.

"Thank you," she said.

Suddenly, she remembered Mr. Matthews didn't know the situation of her birth. A fear overcame her, one that he might no longer respect and admire her if he did. She had no reason to tell him, yet it felt almost as though she were hiding it if she didn't. She'd nearly explained after Belinda's visit, and now it felt as though she should have.

"My mother's and my skills are valued, but we're looked at askance here. I'm illegitimate," she blurted. And it wasn't just her illegitimacy that made her different. It was the circumstances of her conception and the identity of her father.

Matthews went still, just as she'd feared he might. His eyes narrowed, and his words hit a different sore spot, and a surprising one. "They condemn you for your mother's impropriety?"

Anne's temper flared. "It wasn't a matter of choice. She was forced!"

An expressionless mask fell over Matthews's face.

Anne bent her head and covered her eyes. She hadn't meant to tell him that. Dashing away tears, she forced herself to meet her patient's gaze as she explained, "The man who violated my mother is wealthy, powerful, and unscrupulous. When Mum denounced him, she was unmarried, eighteen, and pregnant. He convinced everyone that she lied in an act of desperation. Said Mum concocted the claim of rape to excuse her pregnancy and salvage her reputation, and named him as her perpetrator because he was rich and wouldn't miss the money she hoped to extort from him. It was her word against his. Everyone was appalled that Mum would fabricate such a heinous charge, but the man urged them to forgive her. He said she was young and unwisely thought accusing him would excuse her unmarried motherhood. The swine. It wasn't enough for him to be thought innocent, he had to appear kind and forgiving as well."

Anne had to stop, breathe, push her fury down. She'd learned to do so, to control the rage, but from the day she understood what had happened she'd never been without it. The anger always simmered there, ready to blaze up whenever she spoke or even thought of the event. Kenton had committed a crime, and her mother had been punished. It was so wrong!

Matthews wore a ferocious frown. "Those who believe your mother lied must now treat her like an outcast. Why did she stay in the village?"

Anne shook her head. "She was young and still learning her trade from my grandmother. Later, when we might have left, my grandparents needed her. Mum stayed for them."

All three had been too proud, Anne admitted to herself. How much simpler life would have been if they'd gone. She herself had considered leaving so many times, and each year the urge seemed to grow. Except, where would she go? And, would her mother come? There was the decision to make about marrying Andrew, too. If she agreed, she'd likely live the rest of her life in Buttermere.

"I'm...sorry," Mr. Matthews said. "For everything you and your mother have borne."

His brow remained furrowed, and she believed him. But she had more to confess.

"It's felt good, you not knowing my history. Not because I'm ashamed," she added quickly, "but because I knew nothing false or demeaning or improper could affect your impression of me. Your regard has been formed based on...my own merit."

Oh, dear. She suddenly felt she was complimenting herself overmuch. And would he think it odd that she'd worried about his opinion of her? She ran her tongue over lips gone dry. "Your not knowing has felt odd, as if I'm hiding something or lying. We're becoming friends, though, and so I want you to be aware of what every other person in Buttermere knows. I might as well tell you. The man who raped my mother was Mrs. Jennett's father, Viscount Kenton."

The surgery's front door bell jangled just then. Anne was grateful, actually. Without having to speak of her parentage any further, she pushed to her feet and went to see who had arrived and what help they might be needing.

Nancy Blythe stood just inside the front door, in the small sitting area where villagers could wait their turn, clutching *Sonnets from the Portuguese* against her pregnant abdomen.

"Did you love it?" Anne asked, accepting the slim volume from one of the few townsfolk she considered a friend, the mother of the very first babe she had ever delivered entirely on her own. Anne would never forget Robin's birth. It had been a momentous first for both eighteen-year-old Nancy and fourteen-year-old Anne, and the beginning of their friendship.

Nancy was smiling. "I read it four times! I think Walter was a bit jealous. He kept asking, 'again?' every time I opened it. Except...then I read a bit aloud."

Anne laughed, because quite suddenly the woman's face had turned bright red. "I'm glad you enjoyed it. I knew you would."

"I intend to purchase a copy," Nancy said. "Mrs. Browning very eloquently expresses my feelings for Walter when I take time from my housework and children and"—she paused, looked down, and smoothed a hand over her large belly—"and plans for the future to think of him."

"Here," Anne said, extending the book in a sudden feeling of necessity. "You keep it."

"What? Oh, I couldn't," Nancy said, even as she took the volume and pressed it to her chest.

"I want you to have it," Anne insisted. "Lately it makes me sad when I read it. I've never felt passion like that, and I'm beginning to think I never will."

Nancy squeezed her arm. "Don't give up," the woman urged. "Perhaps, given more time..."

"I don't think my affection for Andrew will ever grow into *that*," Anne said, tapping her finger against the book cover.

Nancy's mouth firmed. "Then, make some changes. I don't want to see you leave, but you deserve to know that kind of love. All of us do who are good and kind and dutiful. It's one of the few rewards we can find in this life."

Yes, but what if I leave and never find the right person? Anne found herself thinking. There was a good man and a good life for her right here. Was she seeking a reward beyond her just deserts? Still, for a moment she couldn't stop thinking of Mr. Matthews and the awareness and attraction she'd felt for him only minutes before.

"Life is short," Nancy continued. "It seems like yesterday when you delivered Robin, but he's already half-grown."

Anne glanced at Nancy's protruding abdomen. "How are you feeling?"

"Well enough. I thought the walk might do me and this little one good. Your mum examined me yesterday. She says I'm healthy and the babe will come when it's ready." She stepped back. "But now I'd best be on my way. I'm sure you're busy, given you're caring for that injured traveler."

"Yes," Anne agreed, "and I'd best make certain pain hasn't kept him from his nap." Indeed, she hoped Mr. Matthews was deep asleep, so they didn't have to discuss her parentage any more today.

She and Nancy said their good-byes, and Nancy left. When she checked, Anne found Mr. Matthews asleep, which made her breathe a sigh of relief. She propped open the front door to prevent the bell ringing when the door swung, and tacked a note outside: QUIET, PATIENT SLEEPING. There weren't any patients scheduled to visit the rest of the day, but a couple of yesterday's had been instructed to return if their condition worsened.

Feeling she'd done everything she could, Anne headed to the kitchen and her lunch.

CHAPTER EIGHT

The following day Peter felt more himself. The Scottish pipe band in his head hadn't stopped playing but was at least marching away, the sharp rat-a-tat of the snare, deep thump of the bass, and drone of the bagpipes somewhat receded. New blossoms decorated the hydrangea bush outside his window, and he actually looked forward to eating. All definite improvements.

Mrs. Pettigrew served his breakfast and remarked that today was Anne's half-day and she wasn't expected until afternoon. Too bad. He'd fallen asleep after their conversation yesterday and hadn't awoken until after she left. After sleeping through the night as well, Peter didn't feel the least inclined to nap. He was wide awake with nothing to do but consider his situation.

By turns, Owen Weaver and Bellow Hill, Arthur and Belinda, and Anne each filled his mind—Anne most of all. Yesterday, when she had explained her parentage, guilt had made his belly flip. Not revealing he already knew her history had made him feel deceitful, but he couldn't let her think he'd gossiped about her either. Ever since Arthur told him, and knowing Kenton as well as he did, his belief had gradually diminished in the possibility her mother was truly raped, but listening to Anne, so forthright and sincere, her clear amber eyes imploring him to understand, he knew *she* believed in the crime to the bottom of her soul.

His thoughts were interrupted as Carter strode in carrying a chessboard and a small box. "Fit enough for a match? Anne suggested you might want to play, and I have no patients at the moment."

"More than ready to turn my mind away from my worries," Peter agreed. "I hate not being able to *do* things."

Carter helped him sit forward, stuffed pillows between the headboard and his back, and ascertained Peter was comfortable. His chair pulled close and the board between them on the bed, he then opened the box and began setting up chessmen.

"Your surgery has been quiet as a church today," Peter remarked. "No comings and goings to eavesdrop upon."

"No," Carter agreed. "I catch up on my bookkeeping on Anne's half-day." The board set up, the surgeon extended his arms and fingers in a long stretch. "I'm more than ready to engage in a bit of recreation."

After a dozen moves and two captures each, Carter chuckled. "It appears we're pretty evenly matched."

"Do you play often?" Peter asked.

"Mr. Jennett gives me a game now and then."

"Who usually wins? Should I accept if he challenges me?" Peter inquired. The surgeon's answer would serve as a predictor of which of them would win this game. Peter and Arthur were fiercely competitive, evenly matched, and each loved lording a win over the other.

"He wins the majority of the time, but not always. This is enjoyable. I don't often have the pleasure of facing a new opponent."

One side of Carter's mouth was tipped up, as if he already believed he'd win. Peter suppressed his own grin. The good surgeon was skilled enough that he needed to pay attention, but he was fairly certain Carter wouldn't be victorious.

Which of them held the advantage switched back and forth as the game progressed, but the final move was indeed Peter's. Carter collapsed back against his chair with a breathy groan.

"That sounds like the end of a hard-fought battle."

A slim blonde woman stood in the doorway, an empty bag folded over her arm. Carter sprang to his feet. "Good morning," he said. "You haven't met Mr. Matthews, have you?"

"I have not," the attractive lady said. She looked at Peter. "How do you do?"

"This is Mrs. Albright," Carter said.

Albright? It took a few seconds for Peter to come to his senses. The woman hardly looked mature enough to be Anne's older sister, let alone her mother.

"I'm pleased to meet you, ma'am."

"Since I planned to stop by, Anne asked me to bring you something," the woman said, moving forward and holding out a pair of tablets, one pocket-sized, the other larger. Peter took the sketchpads and set them atop his little side table. Then Emma Albright delved into a pocket and withdrew a pencil and a ruler. Her fingers, extending the utensils, had the same shape and graceful, assured way of moving as her daughter's.

Peter took the pencil and ruler and placed them with the tablets. "Thank you."

So, this was the woman who'd shared some type of sexual union with Kenton, and who'd accused him of rape. She was lovely, with bright, direct eyes and a soft, sweet face, though a less animated one than Anne's. Comparing her to Kenton's wife, Claire, was like comparing spring sunshine to the crisp notes of fall. Viscountess Kenton had sharp eyes, a patrician nose, and regal posture.

"Is there something you need?" Carter asked.

"Yes. Shepherd's purse and motherwort, please."

"Certainly," the surgeon said, and he ushered the woman out to the treatment room, where his apothecary cupboard stood. Peter relaxed against his pillows and listened. He heard the slide of a drawer and the snap of cupboard doors.

"That's plenty," he heard Mrs. Albright say.

"Any of your patients experiencing problems?" Carter asked. His voice had a different tone than Peter had heard before from the man.

Something more personal, more solicitous. He cocked his head and listened further.

"I'm here any time you need help. Even if you only think there *might* be a problem."

Peter remembered introducing Louisa to his parents, and the next day asking what they thought of her. His mother and father had locked gazes. Waiting for their verdict, he'd felt the way Carter sounded: anxious and uncertain and filled with hope. Today, just as Peter had so long ago wanted his parents to like his potential bride, Carter wanted Anne's mother to like him. To think well of him. Not his medical skills, but *him*. And why else but because Carter planned to become her son-in-law?

Of course that was it. From the beginning Peter had thought the two perfectly matched, like Louisa had been perfect for him. Obviously the surgeon was protecting Anne's reputation in claiming to feel no more than a brotherly connection. Carter was likely the reason Anne had refused Snow; the surgeon hadn't yet asked for her hand. But clearly she was hoping. It only made sense. She was kind, generous, and beautiful, and a dedicated nurse; she'd said the job fulfilled her as nothing else in the world, and the two could only improve their already excellent partnership. Carter could look the world over and not find another woman as suited. The only real mystery was why he wasn't openly courting her.

Peter suddenly felt as sour as Dickens's Scrooge and as bitter as Melville's Ahab. Comparing Carter and Anne to himself and Louisa was...unsettling. Usually when he thought of Louisa, her face came to mind with a wave of pain. Today, no other face but Anne's materialized. It was strange, this sudden absence of sorrow and new attraction, and even more discomfiting to know the object of that attraction was meant for someone else.

"Goodbye, Mr. Matthews."

Anne's mother was back, her bag knotted and dangling from her hand.

"Good day, Mrs. Albright," Peter responded. "I'm glad we had the opportunity to meet, and I congratulate you. You've raised a fine daughter. I'm grateful to her and to Mr. Carter here for my life."

"Thank you," she said. Her eyes glinted, and Emma Albright gave a huge, gleaming smile that offered unfettered pride and happiness and appreciation. Which got Peter thinking. A mother's influence on a child was great. If Mrs. Albright were a selfish liar, would Anne have become such an honest, warm-hearted person?

He looked at Emma again. If he weren't privy to her history, he'd trust that face. That clear, steady gaze radiated openness and honesty. He couldn't imagine this woman making the heinous accusation of rape unless it was true. Nor could he conceive of this face being that of a woman who would seduce a married man. Might she have been tremendously different as a young woman? If she had lied, she'd thereafter chosen to stay and continue deceiving everyone. That sounded like a recipe for a miserable life.

Not that telling the truth—if it had been the truth—had made things much easier.

Peter shook his head, unable to come to a conclusion. Could his godfather be altogether different than the man he believed he knew? If this lady's claim were true, Kenton was worse than despicable. That just didn't seem possible either.

"Mr. Matthews?" Mrs. Albright prompted. He'd been lost in thought, and apparently she'd called his name more than once. He rubbed tension from his forehead, which felt creased.

"Yes?"

"You may see me again before you leave; any number of errands cause me to stop by. In addition, the times when Mr. Carter must be gone at night and there's a patient who needs looking after, I stay. I just wanted you to know."

Peter didn't want to contemplate a circumstance where he might need constant nursing, but he gave a nod. He liked knowing Anne wasn't here in such situations, that she was replaced by her mother, whose age and motherhood—and perhaps, already tarnished reputation—gave her the freedom to do so.

"I hope I won't be the cause of missed sleep, ma'am," he said.

Her head tipped to the side, and she considered him. Then she nodded, said a final farewell and left.

Peter lay in bed, more confused than ever. Meeting Emma Albright had given him an altogether different impression than he wanted. He'd sensed warm-heartedness and honesty, and she appeared youthful enough to be mistaken for an older sister of Anne's, at most a decade older than Carter. And Kenton had either raped or conducted an adulterous affair with the woman?

Neither scenario was believable. Yet one of those alternatives had clearly occurred.

Shortly after the woman left, Carter entered and informed Peter he was walking down to Danvers Retail; Peter had only to call out for Mrs. Pettigrew if he needed anything. Peter didn't, but perhaps ten minutes later he heard the front door open and a woman's lighter steps. His heart raced as he thought it might be Anne who would appear in the doorway, but it wasn't.

It was Belinda.

"Hello, *Mr. Matthews*," Arthur's wife said as she briskly advanced into his room, dragged the chair over to the small table beside him, and pulled paper and pen from a bag that hung from her arm. "Arthur said you needed to dictate a few letters and asked me to scribe them."

Peter opened his mouth to greet her, but she immediately turned and whisked herself back to the treatment room. A moment later she returned with an inkwell and sat down.

"Hello," Peter said. His cousin had stopped by again yesterday evening, which was when Peter had mentioned the need. He'd tried writing for himself but found it painful. "This is kind of you. Where are the children?"

"At Pennyton Park." Belinda glanced toward the door. "No one working today?"

"Mrs. Pettigrew is in the kitchen."

The rigid stiffness of Belinda's spine eased and her chin dropped. "Well. Let's get to it, shall we? I can't be away from Rebecca long."

Of course she couldn't. She'd still be nursing.

"Well…?"

Belinda waited, drilling him with impatient eyes, and Peter found himself apologizing for adding another task to her day. Perhaps this additional chore was too much of a burden in an already busy life—or perhaps Belinda was just in a funk that she couldn't or didn't care to hide. Either way, Peter didn't want to add to her difficulties. In future he'd make sure Arthur did his scribing.

He began with his most pressing need: the letter to his estate manager, informing Aycock of his circumstances and how to address any necessary correspondence to him here. A couple of times he paused to ask Belinda if he were going too fast, but she shook her head and continued to write. As they finished, on a sudden whim he asked her to add, "Please send the following books from Treewick Hall's library," and he rattled off the titles of his three most comprehensive volumes on architecture. The last time he'd opened them, he'd been at Oxford.

Could following that old dream really be as simple as Anne believed? He no longer felt duty-bound to abide by his father's traditional standard for a Viscount Easterbrook. His father hadn't been here to see it, but Peter had proven himself. With the exception of Bellow Hill, which he hoped would soon be fit to resume production, Easterbrook properties and enterprises were sound and no longer required his unconditional attention. But, an architect! Did he still harbor the necessary desire; could he unearth his buried dedication for the study and practice required? Tingles raced down his spine, but he didn't voice his excitement to Belinda. Instead, he turned back to the task at hand.

His second missive was similar to the first, except it was to his man of business, and Peter directed Nickerson to investigate the financial health of Richard Hardesty, his Bellow Hill partner. Hardesty had been eager to link himself to Peter with the investment at the start, calling him brilliant and every modern young businessman's ideal, agreeing to every stipulation without complaint. The colliery *had* been a good investment early on, and Hardesty benefited greatly, but when modernization and the need to improve worker safety impacted his pocketbook the man's attitude changed. Now Peter wondered if the flattery had been pretense or, without Peter knowing it, Hardesty's financial situation had changed.

Could the man be desperate enough to resort to murder? The last time Peter saw him, the seething Hardesty had growled, "You'll be sorry," in an ominous voice, but Peter had assumed he only referred to lost profits. He just didn't see the man as violent.

Belinda flicked a look at Peter as he dictated the last part, but she didn't comment.

The person Peter was most anxious to hear from was the recipient of his third letter, the engineer George Lawton. *Please let him be close to a solution*. By now, Owen Weaver would be in Cliff Gate and would have met with Lawton and Hardesty both. Peter expected Weaver's initial assessment of Hardesty soon, along with details of any miners making threats, and of those absent from the village on the dates of Peter's London attacks.

Belinda took a big breath after the final valediction and laid down her pen. "Arthur will post them tomorrow," she promised.

"Thank you," Peter said. Then, hoping to learn what was causing her such grief he said, "Can you stay a while?" He would do anything to help Arthur be happy again.

Belinda was busy folding letters and placing them in her bag, and she paused. "A few minutes. I prefer to avoid Miss Albright whenever I can."

Ah. Perhaps that explained her taciturn mood, and the mood Arthur had suggested was now so constant for her. Perhaps she was feeling all the confusion and anger that Peter himself felt upon hearing the news. She'd have better cause for it. "Arthur explained."

"Yes. He told me he had." For a moment Peter was pinned by her gaze. "You're close to my father. You had no idea?"

"Of the accusation? I'd heard nothing! Do you believe—?" He stopped. He couldn't ask *that*.

"No," Belinda snapped. Her cheeks blazed. "Father did not assault Emma Albright. I meant about the rest."

He'd put his bloody foot in it. The tightness of Belinda's mouth made her look like she'd swallowed something inedible, so he quickly said, "It must be uncomfortable for you, living and working in the same village as Miss Albright and her mother."

Belinda's head tipped to the side, and she studied him a long moment. Then she gave a surprising answer. "I knew what to expect, and I love Arthur. Not marrying him would have been far worse than living with the ostracism every day."

"Ostracism?" Peter was confused. "By the Albrights, you mean?"

"By the entire village," Belinda snapped. "Arthur doesn't know how bad it is. I don't complain, but they all resent me. My aristocratic birth, my upbringing..."

Ah. *That.* Peter was struck by the irony of both Anne and Belinda being treated like outsiders here, though for entirely opposite reasons. He couldn't help asking, "Do they believe Emma Albright, do you think? Has the accusation toward your father affected you?"

Belinda snorted. "Hardly. Father's a huge benefactor to Buttermere. They're not going to speak ill of him."

What an odd way to phrase the denial, Peter thought.

"I've done my best to be a part of this community, yet I'm barely tolerated. I care for my house and my children myself, and anytime someone needs help—from the poorest families to the well-off--I'm there, helping. They accept it, too. I cook, I clean, I wipe snotty noses, but they thank *Arthur*, not me, and they act as if my efforts are second-rate."

Belinda's eyes blazed. Peter had never seen her like this: angry, and obviously quite resentful. To be honest, he'd never seen any well-bred woman like this. He wasn't sure exactly how burgeoning young ladies of quality were taught to restrain their emotions, but taught they were. So well in fact, he'd never seen a lady lose her temper. Not even his mother the day he decided to burn a wasp nest he'd found and accidentally incinerated a garden shed and her most prized rosebushes.

He supposed he couldn't be too surprised. This life was a lot to ask of Belinda. Before her marriage she had never cooked a meal, scrubbed a dish or a dress or a floor. Servants had done all for her, as they did all for him when he wasn't away on a mountaineering expedition, the one place he escaped the circumstances of his birthright—apart from lying wounded here. He supposed that some of Belinda's bygone servants, hired as extra help when Kenton occupied Pennyton Park, might even still reside in Buttermere.

"I'm sorry it's been difficult for you," he said, not knowing what else to offer. "To be Arthur's wife."

Belinda's eyebrows squeezed together. "It's not Arthur," she said. "It's…it's this place, these people. They're trying to punish me for marrying him. They love him and they don't think I'm good enough for him."

That didn't make sense. Arthur was a gentleman, but Belinda was the daughter of a viscount. Why would they think *her* unsuitable? Even if they did, why would they punish her?

She flung out her hands in a gesture of frustration. "I do everything Buttermere wives do, and I'm a competent—no—an *exemplary* wife."

Peter's eyes went to her fingers. In spite of her claim, the hands Belinda extended were pale and soft, the nails clean and evenly trimmed. The elegant hands of a lady. He wondered how she'd managed to keep them so.

Over the years he had gotten a pretty clear picture of the area from Arthur's letters. This was a small village, and its people weren't wealthy. Most couldn't afford a cook or housekeeper. They did hire a village lad or girl for help, sometimes. Girls helped their mothers with household work and sometimes earned extra pennies by hiring out to do the same for a neighbor. Boys too young for other work swept and blackleaded ovens, cleaned ashes from the fireplaces, and sifted the ashes for cinders. But the majority of the cleaning, laundry, and cooking was left for the matron of the household.

"Do you have help—aside from the usual girl and boy?" Peter asked.

Belinda hesitated. "I could have appealed to my father and obtained regular domestic help, but I haven't. I do everything expected of a clergyman's wife."

Did that mean she had occasional help beyond that available to the townsfolk? She'd left her children in the care of Pennyton Park servants today, so yes, definitely some. Belinda might think she'd earned the right to be included in the collective of Buttermere wives, but her educated speech, her refined way of dressing, her manner of correctness—they all set her apart. And that was how it would always be.

"They don't understand a man like Arthur," Belinda snapped. Face fierce, she leaned forward. "He needs better than the type of wife they all aspire to be. I'm perfect for him. No one could love him more."

Peter had never doubted that. So of course she was unhappy if she felt she was failing him.

"They're jealous," he suggested. Except, if she was truly generous and friendly, they couldn't *all* be jealous. And suddenly he remembered how Belinda had treated Anne the other day.

His cousin's wife bent her head. "I don't want to tell my mother about this, and I can't tell Arthur. You and he are close. I know you'd do anything for him, just as I would, and I thought you should know..."

She didn't finish, but he recognized her pleading tone, pleading for him to understand. But, why couldn't she tell her husband all this? Arthur already knew she was unhappy. He needed to understand why.

"Belinda, you need to tell him how you feel."

Her head jerked up. "Don't you dare tell him. Any of it. Promise me."

Peter hesitated. Arthur was sick with worry, and maybe he could help Belinda effect some change. For a moment the two of them stared at one other, before, with a jolt, Peter realized Belinda's eyes were amber like Anne's. Like Viscount Kenton's. Another reminder of what had occurred all those years ago.

"I won't tell him unless something happens that compels me to," he agreed, compromising that much. He doubted Belinda was so unhappy she'd do anything drastic like running away. No, she loved Arthur and her children too much. So he didn't have to worry that his silence would end in some horrible action he should have prevented.

Belinda stiffened. "I shared this in confidence."

Peter kept his gaze steady. He wasn't yielding more.

Belinda waited, her face flushed, then gave an annoyed huff. "If you *must* tell Arthur, I ask that you tell me beforehand. So I can do it."

Peter gave a short nod. Fair enough. That was what he'd prefer, anyway.

The stiffness of Belinda's neck and shoulders eased. She rubbed her fingertips up and down her forehead and said, "It will all be fine. It *will*."

"Arthur is a man of God," Peter reminded her. "He can help you with this."

Belinda pressed her fingers to her mouth. A moment later, she surged to her feet and picked up her bag. "I need to fetch Rebecca. Good-bye. Arthur should stop in later."

Peter's own farewell was offered to her rapidly retreating back.

CHAPTER NINE

Three mornings after her half-day, Anne found Edwin restocking his bag before setting out on home visits. It had been nine days since Mr. Matthews was shot, and today their patient was taking a turn for the worse. He wasn't sweating, but when she'd checked his forehead with her palm his skin had felt warmer than it should.

"I'm worried about Mr. Matthews," she said. "I think he's developing a fever."

Edwin's shoulders slumped. They had been hoping this wouldn't happen, but there had always been a danger. "How does the wound look?"

"There's an area of redness the size of a plum," Anne said. "He has increased tenderness, but no exudate or swelling."

Edwin's mouth flattened. "Infection. But maybe we'll get lucky and he'll fight it off. I'll take a look when I get back. Use the white willow bark tincture if you need to."

Anne nodded. The tincture, used for fevers, would help wound tenderness, too.

"How many home visits do you have today?"

Edwin closed his medical bag and gripped its handles. "Five. Two out at the mine who sound like pneumonia. You?"

"There's only Mrs. Cooper's burn dressing. This is probably the last time I'll need to see her. She's healing nicely."

Edwin nodded and headed out. Anne followed him to the kitchen, where he stopped to speak to Mrs. Pettigrew. After collecting a custard she returned with the snack to Mr. Matthews, whom she found asleep. There was no denying the flush on his cheeks. She set the custard down and settled her palm against his forehead, and it was hot. Not scary-hot, but intense enough that worry began to chew like pesky midges at the edge of her confidence.

His eyelids lifted, and his eyes scanned her face. He had a nine-day beard now, and the dark facial hair made the blue of his irises appear even bluer.

Anne started to lift her hand away, but he clapped his atop hers.

"Please don't move those cool fingers. They feel so good."

She let her hand relax. His mouth curved and he sighed, and Anne wanted to do the same. What was it about Peter Matthews that made her clench so deep inside? Certainly he was handsome, but it wasn't just his looks that made her ponder what it would be like if he ran his hand up her arm, drew her down to him and kissed her; something far more profound was at play. Something she'd been trying to push away for the past three days, since she'd foolishly told him the truth about her parentage.

Anne forced her mind back to her nursing duties. Before she could ask how he felt, though, the bell on the front door jangled.

"Someone's here." She drew her hand back and headed into the surgery.

William and Delia Snow, Andrew's parents. The pair had advanced through the waiting area and gone into the treatment room, Delia's hand clamped on her husband's arm. William's heavy boots shifted as he attempted to keep his balance; blood saturated the collar and shoulder of his shirt and covered his hands, and the side of his face was smeared with it. A laceration split one eyebrow.

Anne sighed. It had been six months since Andrew's parents had shown up like this, and still that wasn't long enough.

William jerked his arm from his wife's hold, staggered, and caught himself. "Le'go! We're not stayin' here."

"The bleeding won't stop on its own," Delia argued, her words clipped. "You agreed to come." Suddenly desperate, her gaze swung to Anne. "He fell and split his eyebrow. He needs stitches."

Anne looked into William Snow's angry, red-rimmed eyes. His breath smelled of whiskey, and he swayed like a cat's twitching tail. Which likely meant she couldn't reason with him.

Delia sat on the low table Edwin used for patients and patted the space beside her. "Sit here?" she pleaded with her husband, who glared at her.

"Let me just clean the wound and take a look," Anne suggested.

Snow shook his head, and blood spattered the floor. The movement made him lose his balance, too, and he staggered again. He was going to end up on the floor with additional injuries if Anne didn't get him into a chair. Better yet, lying on the treatment table.

Anne stepped forward and took his arm. "Just a quick look."

She tugged gently, but no. He grabbed her hand and jerked it from his arm. Unfortunately, he didn't let go. He squeezed.

Anne raised her chin. "Mr. Snow, let go of my hand." When he didn't release her, she added, "You're hurting me."

Snow leaned forward. She couldn't see a single flicker of understanding in his eyes, and his powerful upper body towered over her, emphasizing how much larger he was in every way. His blacksmith arms, accustomed to lifting and bending iron, bulged, and a sensation like scattering ants filled Anne's arms and legs, hands and feet, leaving a powerful urge for her to run. His eyes widened, and his gaze slowly dropped to her hand, crushed within his squeezing fist.

Only, he didn't release his grip.

"Will," Delia shouted, taking her husband's wrist. "Let go."

She tugged, but he tightened his grasp. It hurt. A lot. Tears blurred Anne's vision. With her free hand, she grabbed Snow's and tried to pry his fingers loose. The pain intensified, and she gasped. Any more and she'd be on her knees. She cast a wild look around. The size of the room, furnished with its two chairs, cupboard, and tables, had never seemed confining, but right now it felt as if it didn't hold enough air.

"Stop," she directed Delia, who still pulled at her husband's wrist and was making it worse. Thankfully, the woman dropped her hands. "Mrs. Pettigrew!" Anne yelled.

From the kitchen, the sound of footsteps coming at a run. Then the cook entered, and she stopped short, skirts swaying.

"Oh, my," she gasped.

"Get Andrew Snow from the stable-yard. Now."

Bless her. Without question or hesitation the cook dashed out the door.

"So, our Andrew's not good enough for ye, eh?" William Snow's upper lip curled, his words slurring. "Ye're a fine one, actin' all hoity-toity when ye're base-born." His eyes narrowed. "Ye need ta be taken down a peg."

Anne hadn't thought his grip could get any tighter, but it did. He was crushing her hand. With a cry, she dropped to her knees.

"William!" Delia frantically pulled on her husband's arm. "Stop!"

Snow's breath heaved. He ignored his wife and kept talking. "Ye're spreadin' yer legs for Carter the same way yer trollop of a mother spread hers for Kenton."

"Let her go. *Now.*"

The voice wasn't overloud, but its grim tone demanded unquestioning and immediate obedience. Peter Matthews stood in the doorway, a pistol leveled at Snow's head, and if Anne didn't know different she would think him fully fit, the way he stood so tall, so steady and threatening. The transformation from patient to protector was almost more than she could comprehend, in fact. He should have looked weak and harmless, rumpled and pale, dressed in his underclothes, and with a bandage wound about his chest, but...oh, he looked so far from it. Instead, he looked like a man accustomed to making hard decisions, acting on them, and not regretting the consequences. A man to be wary of. Snow was bulky with muscle but, of the two,

Matthews was the one who radiated danger. Like heat from a fever. Ferocious.

Relief exploded inside Anne's chest and for one sweet moment obliterated all fear and pain. Her lungs filled, expanded, and she found herself rising up, regaining her feet. Except, Snow didn't react the way any sane—or sober—man would. He didn't release her.

Matthews didn't waste time or words. He stepped forward, and his pistol barrel fixed on Snow's upper arm.

"No!" Delia cried. Her tear-streaked face tilted forward in supplication, she pressed her hands to her mouth and backed off. "Please. He won't be able to work."

She didn't appear to doubt Matthews's intent, and neither did Anne, who moved as far away as she could, pulling at Snow's grip. She should have done so before, because he was too intoxicated to react when she wrenched him off-balance. Except, even stumbling, Snow was powerful. He yanked her off her feet and sent her toppling right into Matthews.

Snow released her hand, and she and Matthews fell. Matthews landed on his back with a sharp cry, and his gun spun off across the floor. Anne went down hard, too, her hip and elbow taking the brunt of the impact.

Snow moved quickly for a drunk man. He picked up the gun and pointed it at Matthews. The next moment his son burst through the door, surprising his father, and grasping the pistol barrel, yanked it away. The father lunged, but Andrew easily avoided him, stepping clear.

"Is everyone all right?" he asked, scanning each of the room's occupants.

"*He's* not," Anne said. Hand, hip, and elbow throbbing, she struggled to her hands and knees and crawled the short distance to Peter Matthews, who lay blinking at the ceiling, face twisted in a sustained grimace. He'd fallen square on his wound, and she felt a brief pang of terror how this might have aggravated his injury.

"He tried ta kill me," Snow blustered.

Andrew exhaled gustily. "Sit down, Father." He pulled William to the closest chair and pressed on the older man's shoulders until his knees gave and he sat. Then Andrew's mouth drooped, his grim expression of anger and disgust giving way to disappointment, his eyes filled with weary resignation.

"The pistol isn't loaded," Matthews said. With a groan, he rolled to his side and pushed up into a sitting position.

Anne couldn't form words. Not loaded? Of course. She should have remembered. The night Matthews arrived, Edwin had removed the charge and placed the empty firearm back in the traveler's saddle-bag. Today, weak and feverish, Matthews had confronted the huge and inebriated Snow with nothing more than his nerve.

"What were you thinking?" she asked.

One eyebrow lifted. "I had to do something. It was the pistol or a pillow."

Anne didn't appreciate humor at times like this.

Mrs. Pettigrew and Constable Weaver burst through the door, and William Snow glared at his son. "Ye sent for the constable? Now ye've done it." He buried his head in his hands.

"Do you need help with him?" Weaver asked Anne, indicating Matthews with a nod.

"I can help," Andrew offered.

Weaver gave another nod and went to deal with Snow.

Anne was already being lent a hand by Mrs. Pettigrew. Back on her feet, she tested her ability to stand, walk, and move her aching elbow. As for her abused, painful, and swelling hand, she was able to curl and straighten the fingers. It wasn't broken.

With Andrew helping, they got Matthews to his feet. The rest she could manage.

"Thank you," she told him and Mrs. Pettigrew.

Andrew turned back to Weaver, his father and mother.

"Do ya see, son?" the older Snow said. "She handles unclothed men, as bold as any harlot. She's not fit ta be yer wife. Ye're lucky she's set her cap for Carter. Only, she's afraid he's too smart ta get hooked, so she keeps ye danglin'."

His intoxicated rant was no surprise, but Anne hated that everyone in the room, including Mr. Matthews, heard it.

Andrew grimaced. "I'm sorry, Anne," he said, then stepped close to his father. "Shut your mouth, Dad."

"I'm locking him up until he's sober," the constable said. "He's caused enough trouble today."

"What about his head?" Delia asked.

"I can't move my hand well enough to stitch it now," Anne said. "It'll have to wait. Take a couple compresses and a bandage roll from that basket." She pointed. "If you can cover the wound and wind a temporary bandage around his head, Mrs. Snow, I'll send Mr. Carter when he returns."

Avoiding Matthews's gaze, she wrapped her arm around his waist and jammed her shoulder into his armpit on the uninjured side. His arm encircled Anne and held tight, and with a moan he leaned against her. Slow and steady, she headed them toward his room. Behind her, she heard the Snows and the constable leave.

"An unorthodox dance to be sure," Matthews joked, "but I'm delighted to partner you. I hope you'll forgive my attire."

He was short of breath and his voice rasped. He was being a gentleman, ignoring Snow's words, and Anne couldn't help but be amused, but right now he should concentrate on walking and breathing, especially when his weakness was so obvious. They arrived at his bed, and instead of sitting and easing himself down, he collapsed onto the mattress. Which must have hurt.

A loud groan broke from him, and he muttered, "My back's on fire."

Anne waited for him to catch his breath and open his eyes.

"Roll to your side. Let me look."

As soon as he was in position, she lifted a corner of his dressing and peeked underneath. The wound was bright red, far redder than it had been that morning, and the skin looked tight. She hoped the change was due to the impact rather than the infection taking hold. After all, under his wound, his scapula bone was broken. The blow had likely cracked every new, healing connection.

With a groan, Matthews settled onto his left side.

"I want Mr. Carter to see this as soon as he returns," Anne told him.

Matthews's breathing had returned to normal. He gazed up at her, his sharp eyes searching her face with admiration. "You were amazing in there."

No. She hadn't been. She hadn't been able to control Mr. Snow, and Matthews had ended up falling on his injury. He'd be justified in blaming her, but clearly he didn't. She couldn't look away, either. Warmth filled her belly, even though she knew she didn't deserve his praise.

"You were so calm," he continued, "and you didn't get angry. You tried to help him. Does this type of situation occur often? One as difficult as this, I mean."

"Not in the same way." Any patient trying to do her harm was rare. She couldn't help but wonder if there had been any way she could have moderated Snow's aggression. When failures like today's happened, she had to somehow turn a disaster into a lesson and go forward. She would be more careful with inebriated patients in future.

Matthews started to reach for her hand, hesitated, then took the edge of her sleeve instead. "Snow said some cruel things to you, but don't you listen. Think instead of how much you are helping the community."

Snow's words indeed hurt. Was *that* what all the villagers secretly thought? But Matthews's reassurances were equally comforting. So often she'd held the hands of others who were hurting, who needed comfort, and today she was the recipient, though the only connection between her and Matthews was the hem of her sleeve.

Below his fingertips, her skin grew warm. Anne wanted to stay just like this and let the warmth of his closeness spread everywhere. To every fingertip and toe, to the roots of her hair, to the center of her heart. But if she didn't withdraw right now, long buried emotions would bubble up and spill over.

The outside door opened and closed. Edwin had returned. So Anne stepped back, said, "Excuse me," and fled.

CHAPTER TEN

Carter's examination of Matthews confirmed the infection was worsening, and whatever knitting of bones had begun, the new trauma had undone. So, after worrying herself to sleep and spending a fitful night, the next morning Anne went in to the surgery early, before Sunday worship, to change their patient's dressing. She planned to examine his wound and determine how he fared before attending church.

First thing, she noticed a change in him. His welcoming smile wasn't as full, and his slow-blinking eyes were bloodshot. This was a very different man from the one who yesterday stood with a pistol in his hand facing an intoxicated blacksmith.

"You didn't sleep," she said.

"Not much," he admitted. "I couldn't get comfortable, not even after Carter dosed me with laudanum."

There was a tightness to his mouth that Anne associated with pain. She set her basket of dressing supplies down and said, "Let's see how your wound looks."

He rolled away from her, onto his side, to give her access. His sheets were damp, and it took no more than an instant of contact with the blazing skin of his back for Anne's heart to sink. She grabbed scissors from her apron pocket, snipped through the bandage and peeled it away from the wound.

Oh, Peter. This isn't good. It was so bad, in fact, she wouldn't apologize for thinking of him with his given name. Yesterday's plum-sized area of redness around the sutures had become saucer-sized and bright red. The area was raised and rounded with swelling, and nasty-smelling pus leaked from the center.

Edwin needed to see this.

"Can you stay on your side?"

"Yes."

But almost immediately he began to roll onto his back. He was even worse than he appeared, if he were too weak to hold himself upright. Anne grasped his shoulder and hip and pushed him back to his side. She'd support him.

"Mr. Carter!" she called.

"It's infected, isn't it?" Peter said.

"We'll see what Mr. Carter thinks."

Edwin strolled in, his pace quickening as he saw them. "Something wrong?" he asked.

Anne raised her brows and tipped her head toward Peter's back.

Edwin bent to get a good look and felt around the wound, grunted, straightened, pressed his lips into a flat line and stared at her. "I need to clip the sutures." He then circled the bed and faced Peter. "It's abscessed. I'll open it up and drain it, then we wait and see." After a moment, he headed into the surgery.

Peter stayed quiet, but Anne knew he understood the severity of the danger. Everyone knew someone who'd died or lost a limb when infection set in after an injury. Opening the wound meant he'd be left with a prominent scar, but that wasn't what mattered. His life mattered. When his eyes closed, her chest filled with sticky heaviness. She gave his arm a gentle squeeze. His eyes opened, and she saw gratitude there. He acknowledged her encouragement with a drop of his eyelids and the smallest of nods; then she tucked several pillows against his chest and curled his arm around them.

"Rest against these. They'll help keep you on your side."

If only he hadn't fallen on his wound. She very much feared it had exacerbated everything. Which was all her fault.

Edwin returned with forceps, scissors, surgical pliers, and lint. After cutting and removing the sutures, he handed Anne the lint, saying, "I'm going to express as much of the pus as I can. When I'm done, you can wash and pack the wound. Do whatever you can for the fever." He leaned over Peter's back and eyed his face. "This is going to hurt."

Peter fisted a handful of bedsheet. Anne circled to the other side and edged forward until her knees were flush against the bed. Her body would bolster the pillows, and she steadied Peter's shoulder and the crest of his hip with her hands.

Edwin inserted the surgical pliers and spread them a couple times, widening the mouth of the wound. Peter tensed but said nothing. Edwin put the pliers aside and pressed against Peter's back, dragging his fingers from the periphery of the redness to the wound opening. Pus spewed out. Peter's body went stiff, and he pressed against Anne. Still he said nothing. Then sweat broke out on his forehead, and a choked sound emerged from his throat. Anne wanted to hug him, to dry his face, to whisper words of encouragement in his ear, but she instead supported his body and handed lint to Edwin.

Edwin explored the wound with the forceps and expressed everything he could until nothing but a thin trickle of pus-free blood came from the wound. Then he nodded, patted Peter's arm, and spoke to Anne.

"I'll be on my way if that's all right. More still to do elsewhere." The surgery was closed on Sundays, making their workday a shorter one, but still there were patients who needed visiting.

Anne nodded and took over. Edwin gathered his medical bag and left.

"We're almost done," she murmured to Peter.

His body slackened as he released the contracted muscles he'd held tight, and the tension in Anne's chest eased in response. She cleaned around the now open wound and packed it with a strip of linen rinsed in silver nitrate solution, all the while maintaining a constant stream of chatter to distract her patient.

"I'm giving you a dose of pain tonic, and you'll drink several cups of water and broth, even if you don't want to. You're to lie on your side to keep pressure off your back." She peeked down at his face, where his mouth tilted slightly upward at the corners. "I'm also giving you white willow bark tincture, then I'm bathing you and fanning you until your fever drops."

Only time would tell whether the infection had spread to his blood. If so, only a miracle could save him.

She finished with the wound. "The rest will be easier if you can sit in the chair a few minutes. I'll help you."

From his silence and the way he avoided looking at her, she doubted he wanted to get up, but he didn't utter a word of protest. Soon she had him sitting upright, medicated and drinking, and she changed the bedsheets as he watched.

"How are you feeling today?" he asked at last. "You took a hard fall yesterday, too."

She sighed. "My hip and elbow are a little sore. They'll be fine in a day or two."

Fetching hot water, she washed and dried his face, chest, back, and arms. She tried to ignore the muscular bulges she slid the washcloth and towel over, muttering, "I didn't realize estate management required so much physical work." Then her hand froze on the curve of his pectoral. *No, no, no.* How could she have remarked on his physique? The stupidity was like lemon juice in a wound.

Peter Matthews took a deep breath, his chest rising and falling under her hand and dragging her back to reality. She jerked her arm away and plunged the washcloth back in the basin of hot water.

"I...climb mountains," he explained.

"You're a mountaineer?" She couldn't hide her surprise. "You mean, on the Continent? Mountains in Switzerland and Italy and... just where do you climb mountains? *What* mountains?" She'd never met anyone who did that. Who had the money and leisure to do such a thing?

"Yes, Switzerland and Italy, Austria and France. I accompanied a wealthy school friend. He...needed a climbing companion and paid most of our expenses."

"Oh." No wonder he'd been so cool, facing Snow with that empty pistol and after being shot on the road to Buttermere. He was accustomed to danger. He must have faced it many times from many rocky promontories. The thought only made more warmth pour through Anne as she began winding a fresh bandage around his chest, adding lots of lint over the wound to absorb any drainage. "What is it like? Have you walked into the clouds?"

"I've been higher than the clouds. It's amazing."

The satisfaction in his voice was palpable, and Anne had no trouble imagining him atop a snowy summit at the pinnacle of the world. "What's the tallest mountain you've climbed?"

"I climbed the Grossglockner. It's the highest peak in Austria."

Austria. How Anne would like to see other countries. To be so high and looking down on the world sounded magnificent, but wouldn't it be harrowing, too?

Finished, she slid around in front of Peter, sat on the edge of the bed, and looked him in the face. She picked up the fan she'd set there, opened it, and began fanning him, using her whole arm to sweep air over his head and torso. "How do you do it?"

"With ropes and special boots and climbing tools."

"No, I mean, aren't you afraid?" The riskiest thing she'd ever done was climb a thirty foot oak to rescue the youngest Elmore child who had climbed up and then been stuck, too terrified to climb down. It had taken every ounce of her courage.

"No," he replied. "It's a lot of things—demanding and exhausting, inspiring and exhilarating—but not frightening. Not the climbing, at least. It gives an incredible sense of accomplishment. Although, on one of my early climbs I lost my footing and fell. That was frightening."

"Were you injured?"

His left shoulder hitched up and down, and he seemed lost in thought. Lost in the memory. "Some wrenching and bruising, but nothing serious. I was lucky. I slid down a steep snowfield. It happened fast, and I had no control. Once I stopped and realized I was still alive, relief overwhelmed me. I starting laughing. I thought Arthur might skin me! I'd scared him, and he didn't appreciate my making light of the situation."

"Arthur?"

"My climbing companion." Peter paused a moment, then continued. "One of the things I wrenched was my ankle. It took us a long time to get down off that mountain. I thought Arthur's teeth would be dust by the time we did." He grimaced. "He told my parents about it. I'd never seen my mother so cross."

Anne raised an eyebrow. "Did you blame her?"

Peter chuckled. "Not really." His eyes squeezed shut and his expression tightened. "Mother would have been within her rights to be ten times angrier. What I'd done was worse than a simple misstep that skirted disaster. Until then, my parents had no idea the level of climbing I engaged in; they thought my rambles were more in the way of scenic foreign nature walks."

"Why was that?"

He paused. "I lied, then for years concealed the truth."

Anne stiffened and quit fanning. She didn't like lies or the people who told them. Disappointment flashed through her. He'd seemed an honorable man.

"You lied out of kindness, perhaps? So they wouldn't worry?" That kind of lie she might excuse, if no one was hurt. Dropping her gaze, she resumed fanning and hoped he hadn't noticed her reaction.

He gave a short, sharp shake of his head. "I began mountaineering as an act of rebellion, and I hid the degree of difficulty I undertook and eventually mastered. I'm embarrassed to admit how selfish and spiteful I was, but during my time on the mountain I was my own man. To my shame, I enjoyed knowing I'd fooled my parents and subverted their control. They'd have been terrified if they'd known."

The guilty timbre in his voice made her involuntary stiffness recede. Somehow, his regret tempered the loathing she'd normally have felt for such subterfuge.

"Perhaps you felt you didn't have a choice?"

He sighed. "Remember how I told you I wanted to design things? When I told him I wanted to study architecture, my father forbade it and insisted I…focus on more traditional subjects. I thought we could reach some sort of compromise but I was wrong. Father refused to bend, which infuriated me. Finally I acquiesced, but I set a condition that university breaks could be spent on mountain rambles. For a long time I was too angry to spend any holidays with them, and on the mountain I didn't have to answer to anyone but myself. And I found I love conquering peaks."

"You resented being forced to give up your passion," Anne murmured, understanding his feelings. "I would have been indignant if my mother insisted I not become a nurse." Still, the situation didn't make a lot of sense. "Why was your father so obstinate? Surely as an architect you'd have a respectable income and be highly regarded? As much as an estate manager."

"Architecture…is a demanding profession," Peter replied. "It can require quite a great deal of travel and not leave much spare time for other projects. My parents wanted me married and settled, doing the traditional work of my father and his father before him." He paused a moment, released a long sigh then added, "Their plan for me was stifling, but at least up on the mountain I was free."

"You came to enjoy your work, I hope?"

"Yes."

"And your parents? Did they accept your mountaineering when you told them the truth?" The breeze from her fan lifted the ends of his hair, and she had a sudden urge to smooth the wayward strands.

"Not exactly. We had an unspoken agreement not to talk about it. When Louisa learned of my hobby, she pestered me for details, and I admitted to scaling the big peaks. Like my parents, she didn't care for the idea of my dying on a snowy mountaintop and leaving young children fatherless. I agreed to curtail my climbing if she'd marry me." He paused. "I haven't climbed since I made that promise."

His expression was contemplative, and Anne thought he was recalling the past—or perhaps he was considering why he still honored that pledge even though Louisa was gone. Anne slowed her fanning then set the fan down and felt his forehead and the side of his face. He was cooler and less flushed. Moist, but not wet with sweat.

His eyes, the blue of the water of Buttermere on a still summer day, studied her.

"I understood why it was crucial to Louisa that I stop climbing," he said at last. "But I don't think she ever understood how important climbing was to me."

Anne had left her hand cupping the side of his face while she thought about his condition. Now she dropped it, his intense regard stealing the air from her lungs. Did that gaze truly penetrate to the heart of her? She felt it there, beyond the shell of her flesh, behind the protection of her ribs, in the place where her dreams, her fears, and her loneliness hid. Those had always been safe, secure from every eye. Until now.

It should have alarmed her. Instead, heat unfurled from her center and spread until awareness hummed through her every cell.

"How do you feel?" Her voice came out lazy and warm as a cat must be, dozing in the sun.

His expression softened. "Better. You've worked a tiny bit of magic."

No. The magic was all on his side.

They both leaned forward the tiniest bit. For the space of several heartbeats Anne hovered, suspended, close enough to see the rim of dark gray that circled Peter's blue irises. Close enough to see every crease of his skin, every whisker. One, two, three heartbeats. His gaze dropped to her mouth. Perfectly synchronized, their lips parted and they dragged in air…

He blinked, and they suddenly both swayed back. That didn't provide enough separation, so Anne sprang to her feet, turned and smoothed the already smooth bedsheets on the bed. Confusion, self-consciousness, and guilt battled for supremacy in her. And, as much as she didn't care to admit it, regret. She'd wanted to kiss him.

"You should rest." She sounded as breathy as she'd been after dashing through a recent rain burst. Felt as exhilarated and alive as she had then, too.

Peter Matthews stood without her assistance, transferred himself to the bed, and stretched out on his side. He said nothing. Anne wasn't sure what to say either.

"We'll leave the covers off unless you become chilled," she managed. Then she busied herself putting the room back to rights.

When next she looked at him, he appeared to be sleeping. Sighing with relief, she headed for a bracing cup of tea and some privacy. She'd missed Sunday worship, but whenever that occurred she felt God understood: A patient's needs came before her own desire to hear Mr. Jennett's sermon and participate in the communal service. She'd spend extra time with her Bible this evening to make up for it. Her mother had missed today's service as well, having been called up to Dale Head Mine to attend the supervisor's missus.

The following hours proved uneventful. Peter slept. Anne restocked and straightened the treatment room then settled into the chair in Peter's room and rolled bandages, all while observing him for any signs of restlessness or the return of fever. Movement at the corner of her eye drew her gaze out the window to see Reverend Jennett approaching the front door. She stood and went to greet him, and waited as he entered the building.

He wrapped his hand around the bell that hung from the front door—to muffle it, she realized. Kind of him. And he was coming after services, which showed a real concern for her patient.

She liked and admired Reverend Jennett, no matter whom he'd married. She'd been beside him many times when a Buttermere resident lay dying, so she knew firsthand how authentic was his love and consideration. In spite of his goodness, however, she never felt comfortable in his presence. She was the bastard sister of his wife and unacknowledged aunt of his children, and there was no escaping that, even if he never mentioned it—because of his kindness or in spite of it, she was unsure.

"Good morning. Is Mr. Matthews awake?" the rector asked in a low voice when he saw her.

"I'm sorry, Reverend. He's asleep."

The man looked disappointed. His visits with Mr. Matthews had featured a lot of laughter, Anne had noticed, so she supposed they were becoming friends.

He fished in his coat and withdrew paper and a pencil. "I'll just leave him a note, then. I promise to be quiet."

"Of course. Please excuse me?" she said, intending to give him privacy and space, but as she started to turn away, his voice stopped her.

"Miss Albright, if you've a moment?"

"Yes?"

"Do you know when your mother might return from the mine settlement? I understand she was needed there."

"She left after daybreak."

Jennett tugged at his earlobe. "It's too early for her to be back, then."

"It may well be tomorrow before she returns," Anne admitted. "Are her services needed?"

With her mother away, Anne stood in as midwife. She hoped that wouldn't happen just now, though. Aside from Nancy Blythe, who was closest, every other woman in the area expecting a baby was a month or more away from her time, and a premature birth was something Anne would rather her mother handle.

"Mrs. Blythe may have entered her confinement. She was feeling unsettled, and my wife was called to the Blythe farm to provide whatever comfort and assistance she could. You haven't heard anything?"

"No," Anne said, as unease twined through her stomach. Nancy Blythe's last delivery had been a difficult one, and Nancy had worried about this confinement since the beginning.

"Well, it wasn't long ago that Belinda left. I told her I'd let you know." The rector drew in and exhaled a large breath. "Let's pray you're not needed."

Anne would send a dozen prayers heavenward.

She left Reverend Jennett penciling a note to Peter and wandered toward the kitchen, where she found Mrs. Pettigrew with an apron covering her Sunday dress, mixing up something in a bowl while a pot simmered on the stove.

"Mmmm. Smells good."

Mrs. Pettigrew's explosion of curly hair quivered as she stirred. "Chicken stew, courtesy of Mr. Cooper. He dropped off a hen in partial payment for Mrs. Cooper's treatment. I'm popping the dumplings on now, so it'll be ready in about twenty minutes. I—"

The sound of footsteps running up the back steps made them both turn toward the kitchen door, then Robin Blythe burst in. The boy stood, legs splayed, breath heaving, face desperate as he cried, "Mrs. Jennett sent me, Miss Albright. She needs your help with my mum. She said to hurry!"

Anne whirled, grabbed the ready medical bag from its wall peg, and ran out the door.

Robin was at her heels. "Take Bess," he said, motioning to his ground-tied brown mare.

Anne hurried to the horse's side and gathered the reins, and the boy gave her a leg up. Astride, Anne found her petticoats frothing around her, her stockings exposed from the knees down. "Don't look," she called to Robin, holding out her hand for her bag. She slung its strap over her head, settled the carrier against her hip, and caught the gaze of Mrs. Pettigrew, who stood on the back porch. "Take care of Mr. Matthews, and let Reverend Jennett know!"

Then she put her heels to Bess and headed for the Blythe farm at a gallop.

CHAPTER ELEVEN

She pressed the mare all the way to the Blythe front door, which stood wide open. Inside Anne found Walter Blythe, who sat in the parlor with his head hanging onto his chest, his hand covering his eyes. His clothing looked as though he'd come from the field: coarse brown pants with braces, a collarless shirt with sleeves rolled halfway up his arms, and well-worn, dusty boots.

He raised his head at her approach.

"I'm here," she said, and the tenseness of his shoulders eased a little. She ran past him to the bedroom, opened the door and dashed inside. There, her heart jumped into her throat and stopped her breath. Then the organ slammed back into her chest and hammered there.

Lord Jesus. Help me.

"Thank God," Belinda Jennett said. She stood at the foot of Nancy's bed, a bundled newborn held securely in her arms, and nodded toward the large puddle of blood pooled under the newly delivered mother. Way, way too much blood. Nancy lay on her back with her nightgown hem at her hips, bare legs sprawled, and her eyes closed. Her hands fisted the nightdress on her abdomen. Tension slammed against Anne's sternum.

Wide and thickly lashed, Belinda's eyes met Anne's and begged for help. "I don't know what to do."

She seemed…angry, almost. Angry Anne was here? Angry that she didn't know what to do? Anne didn't have time to worry about which. Not with Nancy Blythe in this horrible state.

Anne stepped next to Belinda and took a quick look at the baby, just long enough to ascertain its color and breathing were normal. The infant was small but otherwise looked healthy.

She turned to Nancy, bent over her and took her hand. "Nancy? It's Anne. The baby's doing fine. Mrs. Jennett is taking care of…" Her? Him? She hadn't checked if it was a boy or girl. "…the baby. I'm going to feel your womb. See if I can't get this pesky bleeding stopped."

Nancy's eyelids cracked open then blinked. Her gaze slowly sharpened on Anne's face, and her fingers tightened the smallest bit around Anne's hand. Her skin was as pale as a living person's could be. Her lips were colorless, and the blue vein in her temple was readily visible beneath white flesh.

"Anne," Nancy whispered, and Anne heard relief and gratitude and hope in her friend's voice. Her own throat went tight—too tight to reply, so she just nodded and forced the ends of her mouth to move into what was probably a gruesome attempt at a smile.

A pair of scissors lay at the foot of the bed. The ropey blue umbilical cord trailed from Nancy, its snipped end not bleeding but lying in a spreading pool of gore.

Anne released Nancy's hand and placed it at her friend's side. Then she placed her hand just below Nancy's umbilicus and massaged. Normally the womb contracted after delivery of the baby and the afterbirth and stopped any uterine bleeding. A firm, contracted uterus was easy to palpate through the abdomen, but Nancy's womb wasn't firm, and the most likely cause of the soft, boggy uterus and bleeding was a placenta that hadn't completely detached. It hadn't delivered.

Nancy moaned. Eyes gone glassy, she blinked up at Anne, who paused.

"Nancy?"

Her friend's brief rally to awareness seemed to have passed. Anne wasn't even certain her friend recognized her. She clasped Nancy's wrist and found her pulse, so rapid yet faint it was barely perceptible. Her skin was cold, and sweat beaded her forehead. The center of Anne's own chest squeezed and her breath stuttered. Nancy's situation was dire, and Anne was on her own, without Edwin or her mum.

"Did the bleeding start before or after the delivery?" she asked Belinda.

"Right after," Belinda said, voice wobbling. "I've never seen bleeding like this."

Anne increased the strength of her massage, hoping it would stimulate the uterus to contract and push the afterbirth out. Some large clots came, but the womb remained boggy. Blood continued to flow from Nancy, who'd begun to softly cry. Once again, she seemed to have revived a bit and realized something was wrong.

With one hand, Anne kept pressure on Nancy's womb. With the other, she grasped the snake-like umbilical cord and pulled. She'd never done this herself, but she'd watched her mother and knew gentle, steady traction was called for. The placenta was still attached to the uterus, possibly embedded; tearing it away would worsen the already dire situation. She needed to help the tissue effectuate its own release.

The placenta didn't release.

How long should she pull? She didn't know. She maintained the steady traction until her anxiety built to an unbearable level. This wasn't working. She had to try something else.

Stopping, Anne quickly washed her hands at the washstand then dried them on the apron she still wore. Belinda, holding the baby, watched. There wasn't a cradle in the room. The baby was a couple of weeks early, and the Blythes hadn't been fully prepared.

"I'm going to need your help," Anne said. "Put the baby in a dresser drawer and come sit on the bed beside Nancy."

"Help you! Do what?"

There wasn't time to mollify Belinda's obvious fear. Anne went to her medical bag, opened it, and located the bottle of dark ergot powder. Ergot, a fungus found on rye and other grains, produced a powerful cramping of the womb. Should she have Nancy drink this and then try pulling the cord again? Or should she try to reach inside the womb, grasp the placenta itself, and peel it away? Dear God, why wasn't her mother here! Anne had never seen this done. She'd heard it described as something like separating an orange from its peel, only you did it from inside the peel while leaving fruit and rind intact. Better to try the medication and internal compression first, and leave the most difficult and risky maneuver for last.

"I need you to help Nancy," she said. Grabbing the cup sitting on the washstand, she shook a good dose of ergot into it, and added water. "Not too much," she muttered to herself as she poured. Nancy might not be conscious enough to easily drink.

Belinda's brows furrowed as Anne stirred the powder and water with her finger. "We need Mr. Carter," Belinda said. "I'm sending Mr. Blythe to get him."

Edwin could only help if they were desperate enough to try something virtually unheard of: surgically removing a hemorrhaging uterus. Such a surgery would be a last resort, and one it was already too late to take, Anne suddenly realized. Assisting him had taught her that. When someone had lost as much blood as Nancy, they didn't survive the additional blood loss that accompanied surgery.

"There isn't time. Edwin's making home visits. Put the baby in a drawer and help me!"

Lips turned down, Belinda stared, eyes glittering, and clutched the baby even closer. She didn't move to help.

A new tension clamped Anne's neck at the base. Her half-sister might not trust her, might be resistant to taking her orders, or simply might be overwhelmed by the harrowing circumstances, but there was no time to sort out Belinda's reason for balking. This wasn't about either of them.

"This isn't about you. Or me," Anne stressed. "It's about Nancy. Now, hurry."

Belinda didn't speak but stepped to the chest of drawers. She slid one open, spent a moment rearranging the contents, and laid the baby inside. Then she turned back to the bed, her hands gripped at her waist, every knuckle white.

Anne motioned her close. "Sit down." She set her cup on the floor and indicated the spot where she wanted Belinda, next to Nancy. Her half-sister lowered herself to the bed like an arthritic old woman, while Anne encircled Nancy's shoulders and lifted her into a semi-sitting position then gave her a shake. "Nancy!" She spoke loud and fast and firm, and gave her another shake. "Wake up, Nancy."

Nancy's eyelids fluttered.

Anne checked Belinda, whose lips had pulled back from her teeth in a grimace. "Hold her up," she directed. "We've got to make her drink this."

Belinda's arms came around Nancy, and she accepted the woman's weight. Anne let Nancy go, retrieved the cup, and held it to the woman's lips.

"Swallow, Nancy. You're bleeding and this will help. Now, *swallow*."

Anne put command into her voice. People clinging to consciousness were vulnerable to strength and persistence. Many would follow strident direction.

She tipped a small amount of ergot liquid into Nancy's mouth and waited. At last, Nancy's mouth and then her throat moved. Relief eased some of the tightness in Anne's chest and stomach, and she sighed and tipped the cup again. "Drink. *Swallow*."

Watching closely, so as not to give too much, too fast, Anne kept tipping. Nancy's cold hand grasped her wrist and Anne's friend swallowed even as her gaze remained unfocused. She stopped once, coughed, then drank the rest.

Anne nodded to Belinda and helped her ease Nancy back. "Stay here. She's going to need you."

Belinda's nose wrinkled as if she'd encountered something foul. Then she huffed. "Let me get her husband. He can do this."

She made as if to rise, but Anne clamped a hand on her shoulder. "*We're* doing this," Anne said. "You're staying right here." Then she bent and placed her lips to Belinda's ear. "Save her husband from experiencing it," she whispered.

Belinda glared but stayed where she was.

Anne picked up Nancy's hand and gave a squeeze. Though she didn't receive a squeeze in return, she said, "I'm going to try and stop your bleeding from inside the birth canal," giving Belinda a look that said, *That's why her husband can't help*.

Nancy was likely too muddled to comprehend her words. Belinda gave no response, either, so Anne moved down the bed. The amount of blood under the woman's hips and between her legs was massive. A large portion of the bedding was soaked through, with big clots and more fresh blood pooled atop the sheet. It was too much, much too much, and renewed urgency gripped Anne.

"Hold her leg. This will go easier if her knee is bent and her legs are apart."

In order to do so, Belinda had to move down next to Nancy's hips and sit or kneel atop blood-saturated bedding. That would consign her pretty gown to the trash heap, and it was clear Belinda was balking. Nostrils flaring, she dragged in a breath.

Oh, blast. Do I have to tug off my own petticoats and toss them over the blasted bedding? Anne wanted to shake the haughty, privileged, *selfish* woman whose eyes were the exact same color as her own. She pitched her voice lower and softer but let the fire she felt fill it. "What I do will hurt. You may need to hold her hips and keep her from pushing away."

Belinda's gaze seemed fixed on the blood.

"And please, Mrs. Jennett, *talk* to her. Reassure her. Comfort her," Anne said. This was usually her own role, on the occasions she assisted her mother with a difficult birth. Her frustration and urgency mounted. They were running out of time as the blood continued to spread. "I can't do this alone."

Belinda's chin stopped trembling, and her lips pressed tight together. Breaths moving her chest like a trapped, terrified animal's, she nonetheless sat where Anne had indicated, and Anne bent Nancy's left knee and pushed her leg up and to the side.

"Hold it."

Belinda did.

Anne sat down opposite her half-sister and closer to the foot of the bed. Watching Nancy, she slid first her fingers and then her right hand into the woman's vagina. The baby had stretched the birth canal, creating space for Anne's hand, and her fist could now press against Nancy's womb from the inside while her left hand squeezed it from above. The maneuver would compress the uterus, applying significantly more pressure than could be applied with both hands atop the abdomen.

But how effective will it be if the placenta remains attached?

She could waste precious time attempting to peel it away, a difficult and perhaps impossible procedure. At the very least this compression should help, allowing time for the ergot to work.

"Nooo!" Nancy's face twisted and her head thrashed as Anne slowly fisted her right hand and pushed, simultaneously squeezing and pressing down as hard as she could with the hand positioned on her friend's abdomen. Nancy clutched at Anne's outer hand and tried to pull it away. She pushed her feet against the bed, but thankfully she was too weak to slide her body away.

"Belinda, grab her hand."

Belinda tried, but Nancy squirmed out of her grasp. Anne used every bit of strength she possessed to keep her own hand clamped atop the womb, as Belinda tried to get a hold of Nancy's hand, which scrabbled at Anne's. Anne's arms shook as she fought to maintain wilting muscle tension, and then Nancy quit fighting. Her last burst seemed to have used the final bit of her energy.

God be praised, the bleeding appeared to be slowing. *Please, let it be due to the compression and not exsanguination.* Anne doubted the ergot could be working yet.

Belinda finally caught Nancy's hand. "It's going to be all right," she was saying. "It's going to be all right." Her gaze locked on Nancy's face, she murmured the phrase over and over. She pulled her handkerchief from her sleeve, wiped her own eyes and then wiped Nancy's brow. "It's going to be all right."

She and Anne waited. The span of a breath. A minute. An eternity.

Anne checked Nancy's face. Her friend's eyes were open, but she wasn't moving or making a sound. All of her efforts seemed to be centered on maintaining her quick, shallow breathing. Was she conscious?

"Nancy?"

Nothing.

"Nancy!"

Anne's heart clenched. Her vision blurred and she blinked, trying to clear the tears away. She released her grip on Nancy's abdomen long enough to deliver a hard pinch to her patient's thigh, but she still got no response. Her friend had lost too much blood, too fast; she'd fallen into a stupor. Her breathing changed, becoming slower, with pauses between each breath, and Anne's hand slid from her abdomen and felt at her groin, one of the places a human pulse was strongest. She found it, but her friend's femoral artery pulsations were too slow, too weak. Giant hands wrung Anne's hope and heart. They had run out of time. Her friend was slipping away.

Anne left her fingers atop the artery, straightened, and withdrew her right hand from the birth canal. "Her heart is slowing," she told Belinda. Her voice cracked on the last word, and she lowered Nancy's leg. "Her body's giving up."

The scent of blood filled her head and a hard metallic taste covered her tongue. A boulder had landed atop her chest, crushing Anne's heart and lungs, and a noose banded her throat. Fresh tears filled her eyes. She didn't blink but let the whole scene blur. This had happened so unbelievably fast. Reason told her that even if Edwin or Mum had been here, Nancy would still have died. Except, reason didn't affect grief or Anne's sense of personal failure.

She kept her fingers on her friend's ever-slowing pulse, knowing it wouldn't be long.

"I'm sorry, Nancy," she whispered.

"You did everything you could," Belinda responded, and for a moment surprise coursed through Anne. Then she accepted Belinda's reassurance, strange as it felt coming from her, and nodded. Waited for another heartbeat or breath that never came.

"She's gone," she whispered, blinking her eyes until Belinda came into focus. Then she stood, went to the basin, and washed her hands.

Behind her, Belinda stood, hands tightly clasped, gazing down at Nancy. In her downturned mouth, in the creases between her brows and at the corners of her eyes, Anne saw her half-sister's grief. Then Belinda gathered up the blanket that had been tossed on a chair, covered Nancy to her chin, and smoothed back her brown hair.

"I'll get Walter," Anne said. She cleared her throat and hoped that when she spoke to him she'd be able to control the weak shakiness in her voice.

The moment she entered the parlor, Walter looked up and stood. Hope fell from his face, and his eyes brimmed with tears.

Anne put her hand on his arm. "I'm sorry."

Walter strode toward the bedroom. Anne did not go. A moment later, Nancy's husband's tortured cry shook the stillness of the house.

A giant screw twisted inside Anne's chest. Time slipped by. She was brought back to herself by the front door opening. Arthur Jennett entered, his hand palming the shoulder of Robin Blythe. The reverend looked at Anne, his eyebrows rising in silent question, but Anne shook her head and the reverend's mouth tightened. He knelt beside Robin and enfolded the boy in his arms. Anne couldn't hear what the reverend whispered, but she saw his mouth moving next to Robin's ear and saw the boy's shoulders shaking. Then the clergyman stood and, with one arm wrapped around Robin's shoulders, guided the lad toward his mother's bedroom.

He paused in front of Anne, who gave the boy a hug, all too aware of his mother's blood on her skirt.

A couple minutes later, Belinda emerged with the baby. The rosy infant was nestled in her arms, fragile and beautiful.

"A girl?" Anne asked.

Belinda nodded.

Anne ran the back of her finger across the baby's velvety cheek. "Etta Daniels has enough milk for two, and her oldest girl is a good helper. I think she would be willing to take the baby for a while. I'll go ask as soon as I leave here."

"Thank you," Belinda said. "Once he's home, I'll make my father aware. He'll provide assistance."

Anne didn't acknowledge the statement. No doubt Kenton *would* send food and coal, and temporary help for the house and fields. Apart from her own, there was hardly a family in Buttermere that hadn't received Kenton's beneficence at one time or another. Anne didn't begrudge Walter Blythe, though. She believed Kenton's gifting was done to keep others feeling indebted to him rather than out of generosity. After Anne's birth, her mum had refused Kenton's largesse, but rather than an act of dignity and righteousness in the face of his crime, her refusal had been viewed by most as the machination of a silly young woman who was egregiously depriving her child.

The newborn mewled. Belinda rocked the babe in her arms and it settled, and something about the curve of Belinda's neck and shoulders made her seem…vulnerable. Anne and Belinda's gazes collided then, and surprise nearly knocked Anne off her feet. Dark emotion filled her half-sister's eyes; they were portals to a deep, endless well of sorrow.

Had Belinda and Nancy been confidantes? No, it wasn't that, Anne decided. During those last harrowing minutes of Nancy's life, Belinda hadn't acted the way a friend would. Still, her grief seemed no less real than that of someone who'd loved Nancy personally. That look in her half-sister's eyes was a true and personal pain.

Anne reeled, off balance. Other than coldness and resentment, she had never been privy to her half-sister's emotions, let alone shared them. The last few years there had been occasions they were needed at the same time, in the same household, and had worked around or alongside each other, but today they'd worked *together*, and Anne saw heretofore unknown aspects of her half-sister: compassion, and a soul-rending sadness Anne associated with great loss. Anne knew the shame, anger, and hurt of growing up as Kenton's illegitimate daughter, but for the first time she wondered if Belinda, the privileged legitimate daughter, had experienced sufferings of her own. Perhaps suffering very similar to Anne's.

CHAPTER TWELVE

Anne and Carter were both gone making home visits, and Peter felt their absence acutely. He was bored, unable to rest, and feeling trapped. Since the onset of the low fever and wound infection yesterday he'd been achy and uncomfortable. He suspected the discomfort would last a while, until he either improved or...got worse.

He tried reading, couldn't concentrate, and gave up. The spider in the corner seemed to be resting or waiting or plotting, of no more use than a picture of itself. He wished Anne were present. She'd promised to begin reading *As You Like It* aloud to him—only three scenes a day, so he might have something to look forward to—and caused him to laugh at the different voices she would use for each character.

Without her, time dragged. Exhaustion weighed him down, yet sleep evaded him. So he wanted to cheer when Arthur arrived.

"You're a welcome sight," he said as his cousin entered.

Arthur sank onto the upholstered chair and sighed, a noise more like a groan of pain than relief. "On my way in, I asked Mrs. Pettigrew to serve tea." His head fell back against the chair and he added, "I'm in need of restoration. I feel like a heap of laundry that's been boiled and dollied and wrung."

Peter peered at his cousin, whose eyes drooped and whose mouth, which almost never failed to offer him a smile, looked grim. "Why's that?"

His cousin took a deep breath and exhaled with force. "One of my parishioners, Mrs. Blythe, died yesterday after giving birth."

Peter's stomach cartwheeled. Anne had been called to attend that birth! Mrs. Pettigrew had told him yesterday after he awakened from his nap. This morning he hadn't thought to ask Anne how the prior day's delivery had gone; he'd been groggy from sleep as she cared for his wound, and she'd been earlier than usual, and quieter.

Arthur's next words emerged like a terrible confession. "Belinda was there through the whole event, and she had to help Miss Albright, which is never comfortable. When we arrived home, Belinda burst into tears."

"You were there, too?" Peter said.

Arthur nodded. "Belinda, Miss Albright, and I stayed with Mr. Blythe and his son Robin until Mr. Blythe's parents arrived. Death is never easy, but Nancy Blythe's is particularly tragic. She left a young family behind. The baby came before Miss Albright arrived, in good fettle, but the mother began hemorrhaging almost immediately. The life just bled out of her." Peter's cousin folded his hands and added, "Before they left, Miss Albright and Belinda cleaned the blood away and put the room and Mrs. Blythe's body to rights, but how do you put a family to rights? During times like these, I'm truly glad I have the solace of God."

The event sounded horrific. How did Anne carry on when a patient died? Especially a death like this: a mother or baby during a birthing.

"Given the small size of the community," Peter remarked, "it must be particularly hard when a crisis or a death occurs. I imagine Anne, you and Belinda are acquainted with every single resident."

Arthur nodded. "Miss Albright and Mrs. Blythe were friends."

Peter wished Anne had shared this with him rather than locking her feelings inside, which was how he now viewed her quiet demeanor this morning. Was she struggling to get through her day?

Who offered her relief in situations such as this? Her mother? Or, as unsettling as he suddenly found the thought, maybe Edwin Carter or Andrew Snow. She'd brought him so much comfort, himself, a strong need to return the favor filled his chest with cotton-wool wadding.

"It's true, there are no strangers in Buttermere," Arthur went on. He frowned. "Although, none of the women have taken Belinda to their bosom. As hard as she's tried, she's never overcome the disparity created by her upbringing."

Yes. Peter recalled Belinda's previous confidence.

"Belinda and Nancy Blythe weren't close," Arthur continued, "but they were on friendly terms. Watching, being part of yesterday's tragedy…it would bruise any woman's heart. Especially a woman like Belinda, who plans to have more children."

"Was Rebecca's birth difficult?" Peter asked, then thought better of it. Once voiced, it seemed a silly and impolite question. Wasn't every birth difficult? Still, Arthur seemed eager to unburden himself, and this prompt might help him.

"No more than average. She didn't want Miss Albright or Mrs. Albright attending her, so Carter did." Arthur paused, clearly caught up in the memory. "I understood, but it made me worry, since midwives are far more experienced with birthing than surgeons. There were no complications, but…well, Mrs. Blythe's death, the how and why of it, is exactly why every woman frets. Even women who've already birthed children without difficulty view the time of carrying and delivering a new child with trepidation. They tend not to talk about how much they fear childbirth, but sometimes they ask to pray with me before the event, which is how I know. I wanted so much to comfort my wife last night, and I tried, but it took hours to calm her. She finally slept, but I stayed awake."

He rubbed his forehead as if overcome, and Peter sympathized with his cousin. He wasn't sure why he thought he could be a better friend to Anne than people she'd known her entire life, but he could barely contain his longing to console her about any and all feelings regarding what had happened yesterday. He wished he had an idea when she'd be back.

Carter's housekeeper arrived, wheeling the tea cart and saying, "I've brought something to tempt your sweet tooth, Parson."

Arthur stood. "You're too good to me, Mrs. Pettigrew."

"That's not possible, Mr. Jennett," the woman said, flashing both men a smile.

"When will Miss Albright be back?" Peter asked.

"She should return around four o'clock. Is there something you need?"

"No, I was merely curious. Some of her days are long ones."

Mrs. Pettigrew gave a nod. "She's a fine woman and a hard worker."

"I've never known finer," Peter said, and congratulated himself on the mildness of his tone.

Pouring their tea, the cook-housekeeper demonstrated she remembered how they took it. She then left Peter and his cousin enjoying individual gooseberry tarts as well, and for a time they ate and drank in silence.

"I'd like to do something to give Belinda ease," Arthur finally said. "A picnic by the lake, perhaps." He tilted his head. "I wonder if Carter would release you for an afternoon so you could join us? The fresh air would be good for you, as long as you didn't overdo, and the weather's been unusually mild. I trust you're fit enough to climb in and out of a carriage?"

Peter certainly wanted to. He'd been almost two weeks in this room. And he *was* feeling better today.

"I think I could manage," he said. "Yesterday Carter opened my wound in order to drain a pocket of infection, but I feel none the worse for wear at the moment. I'll get him to agree, and see if I can't employ Mrs. Pettigrew to provide our picnic fare."

"That would make the outing a special treat for Belinda," Arthur admitted, "having someone else provide the food. Let's aim for Wednesday, then. You'll have another day to heal, and it'll give Mrs. Pettigrew any time she'll need."

"Wait. What are we thinking?" Peter objected, remembering. "Someone tried to kill me. He could be watching, waiting for another opportunity. Our picnic could put you, Belinda and the children in danger. Feeling safe here at the surgery I've stopped worrying about any immediate threat, but it is why I'm here in the first place."

Arthur thought a moment, then shook his head. "I'd know if there were anyone new visiting the area. We needn't worry—unless someone has been waiting in the shadows for the past ten days without making any inquiries about the man found shot on the road! No, I think it's safe to have a short picnic, assuming we keep ourselves to ourselves."

Peter supposed he agreed. Constable Weaver had stopped by and reported he'd warned every farmer to be on watch, and spread the word to Borrowdale, Loweswater, Braithwaite, and Keswick, as well as the smaller villages around them. And ten days was a long time to have heard of no strange occurrences or people in Buttermere or the surrounding farms and towns.

Just before he left, Arthur turned over a letter from Kenton—a missive in response to one Arthur had sent to the viscount's Berkshire manor informing his father-in-law of Peter's situation. Seeing the familiar, strong lines of his godfather's script renewed all the emotion Peter had experienced the day Arthur told him of Anne's parentage, and his chest squeezed with both fondness and fear. He just couldn't fathom Kenton betraying his wife or denying Anne confirmation of his paternity, or denying her financial security. There must be *some* reasoning behind Kenton's actions. Something that explained it.

So...Kenton had broken his marriage vows, but maybe he hadn't precisely betrayed his wife. Anne was in her twenties. No one but Lord and Lady Kenton could know the state of their marriage all those years ago, and maybe they'd come to some arrangement. And Anne was proud and independent, so he imagined her mother was similarly so, so maybe if she'd refused his offer—

No. Kenton was a wealthy man. He should have found a way to provide for his daughter. Insisted.

And *rape*. The allegation alone sent chills down Peter's spine. His godfather, a rapist? This was the man who'd stood by Peter's side, hand on his shoulder, as the bodies of Peter's parents were interred.

The man who'd faced Peter's father and argued that Peter should be allowed to follow his heart. Kenton *couldn't* have raped Anne's mother. He was not an evil man, and rape was an evil act. Peter was certain of that.

He began reading the letter. Kenton's words communicated shock and anger at Peter's circumstances, expressed concern for his condition, and offered assistance. He urged Peter to go to Pennyton Park to complete his recovery. Lady Kenton was already there, and Kenton would join them as soon as his business was concluded.

It was a fine idea. The safest, really. He'd be deep inside Pennyton Park, where a stranger could never get. Certainly that was better than endangering Arthur and his family or anyone at the surgery. Except, Peter couldn't forget the topic of Anne and her mother, and he didn't imagine Kenton would welcome the kind of questions to which he now needed answers. And, how would Anne feel when she discovered Peter and Kenton were close friends and Kenton was his godfather?

Dread settled into Peter's chest, for he knew the answer.

~

Anne stabled Snowflake, the mare Edwin kept for her use, and rubbed her down, watered and fed her, and curried her black, white-dappled coat before leaving Edwin's shed. Smoke's empty stall told her Edwin wasn't back.

She found Peter propped up in bed, pencil in hand. He'd removed his arm from its sling but kept his elbow close to his side, working on the larger of his two sketchpads. It was the first time she'd seen him try it, and a warmth spread through her at his use of her gift. Also, because it meant he must be feeling better than the day before.

He stopped when she entered and approached his bed.

"Are you able to draw without pain?" she asked.

"I have to keep my arm still, mostly just moving my hand. Otherwise, it hurts. It makes these sketches pretty rough, but they help pass the time. It's been a godsend the past few days. *Thank you.*"

Anne fought back pleasure at his gratitude, stepped even with his shoulder and got a good look at his work, which filled her with wonder. "It's Reverend Jennett! You've captured him perfectly." Peter had caught something subtle yet unique to the rector. Humor curved Mr. Jennett's mouth in an uneven smile, and a teasing glint sparkled in his eyes. A laugh burst free as she added, "You talked of drawing buildings, but you're a true artist."

"No. I'm not," he argued. "I enjoy sketching is all. This type of drawing is nothing more than a hobby."

Anne sank into the nearby upholstered chair, which someone—Reverend Jennett, perhaps—had moved closer to the bed.

"You're a man of many talents," she remarked. Peter Matthews managed a nobleman's estate, climbed mountains, and leapt to her defense when barely able to stand. He was particularly solicitous of the welfare of his horse. Now it seemed he was something of an artist as well, and an unreasonably modest one.

She glanced at his face and found those blue eyes gazing back at her. Her heart moving into polka rhythm, her cheeks heated. She dropped her gaze back to the tablet and tipped her head down.

"Are there more?" she asked.

He turned back the page with Mr. Jennett's picture, revealing a detailed drawing of a grand building. The centered dome put Anne in mind of the National Gallery, but this building lacked the Greek facade and columns.

"Oh. This is…amazing."

He turned the page again, and she saw a schematic of the inside of the building, with each story a separate diagram. She studied the many rooms' labels and read the notes he'd penciled in the margins as well.

"It's a museum?"

"It could be," he said.

She held out her hand. "May I?"

He hesitated then shrugged his uninjured shoulder and offered her the tablet. Anne took it, examining each page with renewed disbelief. He'd been sketching a lot. She hadn't realized, as she'd never seen him in action. There was another even more detailed building: a theatre, or opera house, perhaps. Then Mrs. Pettigrew, looking so lively that Anne chuckled. A horse, titled *Red,* made her smile. True, neither the horse nor the people were as finely drawn as his buildings, yet he'd captured their personalities. The sketches were delightful, each in its own rough way.

She turned to the next page and knew exactly who the woman depicted was.

"That's Louisa," he said, confirming her assumption.

Everything faded but the drawing before Anne. Peter's fiancée had been elegant; she smiled with the supreme confidence of a woman admired by all. Fine patrician features, glimmering eyes, and shining, lustrous hair were all portrayed with skill well beyond that of a hobbyist. Or perhaps love had guided his pencil. Peter had even managed to depict the shadow of a dimple in her cheek.

She was serenely beautiful, and Anne dared a glance at the man who had captured her. Eyes hooded, Peter gazed at his beloved's likeness while his thumb stroked across the hem of his blanket. His voice seemed to emerge from a very deep place.

"So many plans...dreams...lost. That night, the night of the accident, I fought to survive, and I lived. But...I lost *everything.*" He paused and took a breath. "I forced myself to go on, to honor the memory of Louisa and my parents. Ten days ago, I again came close to meeting my maker." His eyes blazed. "Sometimes I think God can't make up His mind about me."

A strange hurt built in Anne's chest, like sorrow sharp and cold, a freezing of the spirit. For a long moment Peter held her gaze before studying the picture again, and then finally he sighed. The tension melted from his face, and the lines marking his forehead and scoring the corners of his mouth disappeared. He motioned for her to turn the page.

Anne did, and the air in her lungs froze again. It was a likeness of herself. Clearly it was her, and yet...it wasn't. This woman's hands, wrapping a bandage around a roughly-dressed man's arm, were long, graceful, gentle. Somehow he'd made her face look both determined and vulnerable. The corners of her soft, full mouth tipped up, offering reassurance. The set of those shoulders said she could be leaned upon.

Could the marks of a pencil convey all that, or was she imagining it? It was the only picture he'd shown her that represented a figure in motion, with more than one person involved.

"This...*this* is how you see me?"

It didn't sound like her voice, all high and breathy and thin.

His brows lifted, and one corner of his mouth tipped. "I'm sure it's how everyone sees you."

Her laugh was sharp. "Surely not. You've made me look..." She stopped. She couldn't add *beautiful.*

Though she feared he'd see how deeply he'd touched her with the portrait, she dared a look at him. Not only had he portrayed her as beautiful, but as a woman of admirable character. A warm, vital woman. A woman who could be trusted and admired.

"I tried to show your strength and compassion," he said. His eyes, direct and steady, glinted with an honesty so pure that her heart squeezed. Then he frowned. "Have I offended you?"

"No! You surprised me, is all. The sketch is very complimentary. And...you've far more skill than you give yourself credit for."

She closed the tablet and handed it back before she could blurt out something inappropriate. Before she revealed that his picture made her heart leap. Should she ask him for it? Somehow, even though he'd created it, she wasn't sure how she felt about him possessing it. That picture revealed far more than her mirror's superficial reflection could. It divulged quite a lot about *him,* about how he regarded her, as well. He'd clearly thought a great deal about her while he created the likeness, and the idea of him keeping the sketch, looking at it whenever he wanted, made heat roil through her. Made her chest too tight for easy breathing.

Oh, how silly! As if taking the picture away would remove the intimacy; he had only to put pencil to paper to make another. Then a sudden thought struck her like lightning hitting a tree. What would he think if she requested a drawing of *him*?

"You're the strongest woman I've ever met," he said suddenly. "Discounting our monarch, of course." He started to smile but quickly sobered. "Maintaining such strength must sometimes be difficult. I heard what happened yesterday. I'm sorry."

A sudden image of Nancy Blythe, lifeless, filled Anne's mind. She'd been pushing it out of her mind all day, and she tried once more. She folded her arms and hugged herself, and Peter's capable-looking, muscled hand slid around her wrist. The small connection conveyed unspoken support, and warmth spread up her arm and eased the tension in her shoulders.

"It was a horrible day," she admitted. She had the sudden urge to lean into him, to sink into Peter Matthews's arms. He'd chase away the blame she couldn't shake, and the emptiness.

"How is the babe?" Peter asked.

Checking on the infant had been Anne's first task this morning. "Doing well. Her father named her Nan, for her mother." And Etta Daniels had agreed to take her for the foreseeable future.

"Mr. Jennett was here earlier. He said...he said his wife was deeply affected."

Yes. Anne recalled the sorrow in Belinda's eyes, and the fragile link she'd felt between them. But she couldn't quite bring herself to say that, so she said, "Mrs. Jennett helped Nancy in ways I couldn't. I'm sorry it disturbed her, but such a reaction is understandable." Anne found herself grateful and wanting to help her half-sister now, but how would Belinda react if Anne went to her home? Given what they'd shared yesterday, would Belinda welcome her? Would she find it comforting to commiserate with someone who'd endured the same shocking event? Or would the past always stand between them?

The past. All those years of snubs, those repeated refusals to acknowledge Anne, they all rushed back, sending a chill to Anne's core. No, she couldn't visit the rectory. Belinda's husband was more than capable of easing his wife's distress. Perhaps he was even better suited to it.

"The woman who died...she was a friend?"

Anne nodded.

"I'm sorry. It must be horrible, having a friend's life slip away while you're trying to save her."

Over the years Anne had become proficient at coping with grief, and she allowed herself to remember friends' final moments only in very controlled, manageable doses. She'd been trying not to think of the last endless minutes of Nancy's life, but last night she'd dreamed of her friend's death in great detail. Startled awake, she'd banished every lingering image from her mind. Permitting only tiny sips of pain worked.

Except, when it didn't.

Like this morning, when Etta Daniels placed Nancy's newborn in Anne's arms and love welled up, so sharp and fierce and out of control that Anne almost wept. And all the emptiness she'd refused to feel gouged and gouged and gouged her chest until it felt like a cold, black, bottomless mine shaft. Without heat. Without color. Without light.

Peter waited quietly before her, and she remembered that he had experienced great loss of his own. He'd been at the bottom of that mine shaft too.

"Yes, it can be horrible," Anne acknowledged. "My patients are often my friends—a disadvantage to nursing in a small community. I try not to question God's plan or be angry at Him, and I remind myself that the joyful times are all the brighter for the occasional darkness."

Peter made a noise she couldn't identify, and when she looked up his face was solemn. He said, "We haven't known each other long, but if you're in need of a friendly ear or even a few moments of quiet company, I'd feel privileged to provide them."

A simple offer, and one a friend would make. That mussed dark hair hung over his forehead. Whisker stubble darkened his jaw. The skin beneath his eyes looked bruised, and yet, as rough as he looked, there was nothing about him she found unappealing. Sincerity and deep caring shone from his eyes. And was there more?

He didn't seem to care about the illegitimacy of her birth. He seemed supremely confident and kind, a man who would let nothing stand in the way of him obtaining what he wanted. They were matched in intelligence and station, and he'd drawn that picture…

Why?

A thought, an idea, and suddenly an almost certainty brought her heart and mind to attention: What was growing between them wasn't one-sided. It wasn't ordinary. It was special. So special that she couldn't equate the sunshine filling her chest and radiating out like glowing, unfurled ribbons with the comfortable warmth of friendship. This luminance was nothing short of vibrant, incandescent joy.

Despite her hesitation over accepting Andrew Snow's proposal for the lack of this very thing, she suddenly realized she'd never expected to feel this way or to meet such a man. Not really.

But here he was.

CHAPTER THIRTEEN

The next day passed quietly. Anne ordered medications and supplies and restocked the treatment room as usual, but being near Peter made everything seem brighter: the hydrangea blooms outside his window, Mrs. Pettigrew's rosy cheeks, the burst of sun after a morning shower. Once, when he smiled, she was struck with the notion that he made *her* shine, and she had to leave the room to hide the sudden blush she felt heating her cheeks.

She was sweeping the floor in preparation of leaving for the day when Michael Elmore burst through the front door carrying his five-year-old little brother pick-a-back.

"Let go," he said over his shoulder after staggering to the treatment room and backing up to the examination table.

Anne moved close and unwound Timothy's clenched arms from Michael's neck. The boy released his legs from his brother's waist and sat, giving the table his weight. He was in a bad way. Wide-eyed, pale, and tense, the five-year-old held completely still apart from his wild eyes and straining chest.

Except, his chest wasn't laboring enough. It scarcely moved. Those quiet noises were barely audible, which meant the asthmatic boy's airways had shrunk down past the point of wheezing. He wasn't getting enough air to wheeze. The stiff, upright way he held himself meant he needed every bit of his remaining energy, and every bit of his remaining open lung space, for oxygen.

"Hold on to him," Anne instructed Michael. If Tim lost consciousness, Michael would stop him from falling.

The older boy hopped onto the table and put his arm around his brother, and Anne hurried to the apothecary cupboard. She knew exactly where the canister of dried thorn-apple sat, clay pipe beside it, but tension cinched her stomach as she removed the canister lid and peered in, an involuntary sound escaping when she saw the small quantity of crumbled leaves at the bottom. She'd ordered more but it hadn't arrived.

Enough. It would have to be enough.

Pressing dried stem pieces and leaves into the pipe bowl as she walked, Anne headed for the stove in the reception room. There she fired a spill and headed back to the treatment room. Tim watched as she held the flame to the bowl and drew on the pipe. He'd been through this before, and they all knew what was happening. He needed the thorn-apple as fast as she could get it to him.

With each breath, his shoulders lifted as he struggled to get air into his lungs. He was too weak to hold the pipe, so Anne held it for him. Lips tight around the mouthpiece, he tried to draw the smoke in but it rose from the bowl in a thin curl. His alarmed gaze jerked to Anne.

"Can't. Breathe," he wheezed, hardly loud enough to hear.

"You're going to be all right," Anne assured him. She turned the pipe and put the mouthpiece between her lips, drew the smoke in, then gently and as slowly as possible exhaled it into the boy's face.

Tim nodded. He'd done this once before with Edwin.

Anne wished Edwin, who smoked the occasional bowl of tobacco, were here, but he hadn't yet returned from his routine home medical visits. Each draw of the thorn-apple burned her lungs. She managed to withhold all but the occasional cough, taking small, measured pulls on the pipe. She didn't want any of that valuable smoke going to waste, so she needed to keep her inhalations and exhalations controlled.

Michael pressed his thumb and forefinger to his eyes. Sniffled. "Thank you, Miss Albright," he said, his adolescent voice gruff.

Anne met his gaze and gave a nod. "Your parents?" she asked. Then she drew on the pipe again, pursed her lips and blew another stream of smoke into Tim's face.

"They're being fetched," Michael answered.

She didn't yet see any improvement in Tim's breathing, but his body wasn't quite as tense. The boy's once-fisted hands now lay open. She took one of them in her own, and his fingers tightened around hers.

Movement from the corner of her eye caught her attention. Turning her head as she inhaled, she found Peter watching. He'd somehow managed to don a nightshirt and throw a blanket over his shoulders. Why couldn't she keep the man resting? She remembered when he'd gotten out of bed to help with Snow and ended up falling. She didn't want two patients needing immediate attention.

He walked over, slow and careful. "Can I help?"

She gave him a look of exasperation and blew more smoke into Tim's face. She hoped he'd figure out that meant she wasn't able to converse, and that she wasn't any too happy he was up—especially when she'd heard he was going on an outing tomorrow with Reverend Jennett. But when she tipped her head toward the door, Peter didn't retreat.

"It's bad this time," Michael said. "So bad, Tim couldn't smoke the pipe himself." He leaned closer to his brother and whispered, "He's the man shot on Honister Pass."

Tim's eyes widened.

Peter moved away. Anne felt the edge of a chair nudge the back of her legs, and when she heard, "Sit," she sat, surprised and relieved. She hadn't realized how strained she'd been, standing in that bent position as she smoked, keeping her head near Tim's. A large palm covered her shoulder, and the fingers squeezed. Then Peter moved to Michael's side, leaned his hip against the table, and gave the boy's shoulder a squeeze.

Time passed. After several more smoke-infused breaths, Tim reached for the pipe. Anne handed it over. The child was now able to take slow, steady draws by himself. They were short, but he was getting the smoke down into his lungs. The treatment was working.

A bit of ash glowed in the nearly empty bowl. It would soon be finished. Enough thorn-apple remained in the canister to half-fill the bowl again, but she'd wait before using the rest and allow the first treatment time to work. Maybe the child wouldn't need it.

"You're doing well, Tim," Peter said.

The boy looked at him and gave a relieved smile around the pipe mouthpiece.

Anne, however, was stern. "You'd best return to bed before you end up on the floor, Mr. Matthews."

The smile he gave her was not for Tim, not for Michael, but wholly intended for her, and it burst into bloom something inside that had lain dormant her entire life.

The front door bell jangled. A woman's voice called out, and a moment later Faye Elmore hurried into the room.

"He's better, Mum," Michael said.

Mrs. Elmore turned a questioning gaze on Anne, who nodded. "Much better."

Mrs. Elmore's head and shoulders sagged. She dragged in a breath and gave a choppy laugh, turning to her youngest boy and saying, "You *would* do this the day your father's making a beer delivery to the mine."

Tim, smoking the last of the thorn-apple, shrugged. His mother finger-combed his tousled hair away from his face.

Anne gave Michael a wink. "Mr. Carter is also away, but we managed well enough."

"Of course you did," Mrs. Elmore said. "You always keep Tim—really, all of us—calm. You, as much as Mr. Carter, bring Tim back from the brink. Thank God you were here and knew what to do."

"Thank you," Anne said. Warmth and a feeling of lightness filled her. Gratitude like this was rare but part of why nursing was so rewarding.

"You have two brave lads here," Peter interjected, and Michael and Tim's heads rose like he had draped medals around their necks. Identical grins spread across the boys' mouths.

"You're the man shot on Honister Pass," Mrs. Elmore said, as if she'd just noticed Peter. Anne performed the introductions, adding that the Elmores owned Haystacks Tavern, and then she shushed everyone.

"Quiet while I listen to Tim's breathing."

Carter had taken his stethoscope tube with him, so Anne placed her ear flat against the child's back and asked him to breathe as slow and deep as he was able. After listening to several areas of his chest, she straightened. "I hear some wheezing, but I hear air moving in and out, too. How do you feel?"

"Like I can breathe," Tim answered.

"Good enough to go home, or do you need more thorn-apple?"

The boy shook his head. "I want to go home."

"No chores for you tonight," Mrs. Elmore said.

"Can I have pudding?" Tim asked.

"Yes, love, you can," his mother replied.

"And coffee," Anne said. "A cup today and in the morning. Do you have beans?"

"Yes," said Mrs. Elmore. "I keep them on hand for whenever Tim's chest feels tight."

The two Elmore boys slid off the table onto their feet. They told Peter good-bye and headed for the door, and their mother sighed before saying, "I hope you'll forgive their lack of manners in not thanking you, Miss Albright. Right now, I don't have the heart to reprimand them."

"It's fine," Anne reassured her.

"Normally I'm diligent with my boys, given they're surrounded by bad examples."

"Bad examples?" Anne rubbed at the tightness behind her neck.

Mrs. Elmore darted a quick look at Peter and flushed. "It's a shame, the way some people talk about you and your mother. I've never said it before, but..."

Frowning, Peter straightened and folded his arms. Anne felt her face grow warm.

"I'm sure the maligners don't care to restrain themselves," Mrs. Elmore continued. "I promise, though, that whenever I hear them insinuate something unseemly, I give them a piece of my mind. And others shouldn't believe anything they hear from idle gossipmongers," she added to Peter.

Gratitude fired through Anne, and fatigue. "Thank you," she said, and she reached out to clasp Faye Elmore's hands.

"No. Thank *you,*" Faye responded. Then she gave Peter a pointed look and left.

Silence filled the surgery. Anne drew a breath, forestalling the moment she had to turn and face Peter, face his knowledge of all the difficulties she suffered here. Then he spoke from behind her.

"I imagine the viscount contributes to, or is wholly responsible for, the income of many living in and around Buttermere," he said, moving closer; Anne knew from the way heat flared across the top of her shoulders and down her arms. "It's likely some say what they do in order to assure their security."

Anne half nodded. He was surely correct: Many residents would find it easier and more advantageous to loudly side with the man who managed the parish purse strings.

"I don't mind it as much for myself as I do for my mother," she murmured. "The ones who believe Kenton think Mum's an immoral liar." Anne hesitated then surrendered to a compulsion to reveal the rest. "I feel watched, of course. They wonder if I'm a liar, too, and it's so unfair. To both of us."

"It is," Peter agreed.

Anne turned, surprised. Peter looked like he'd been cracking walnuts with his teeth and was considering cracking a few heads next. She grasped his arm, which drew back so that her hand slid down its warmth and found his, the fingers of which curled around her own. It was just a gesture, but all the same it felt like he cradled her in his arms.

"I'm accustomed to it," she said. "Usually, I can dismiss it."

"It's not right," Peter repeated. "It's just not right."

"It's not," she agreed. "And it's not right that you're standing here this long; so back to bed you go."

CHAPTER FOURTEEN

Wednesday came, the day of Peter's scheduled picnic. Arthur and his family arrived in a carriage bearing the Kenton crest, which surprised Peter, and which he tried not to let show. There was no point in letting on how solicitous he was becoming of Anne's feelings and how torn his own were about his godfather.

"I borrowed Pennyton's clarence so we'd have lots of room," Arthur remarked, helping him out the surgery front door. Anne and Carter did not follow, each having told him to be exceedingly careful if he was set upon such a venture.

His cousin supplied an additional boost, and Peter clamped his teeth together and pulled himself up into the conveyance. In deference to Belinda and Henry, he withheld the curse he wanted to bark. Holy God, but bending over and stepping up into the carriage hurt—more than he'd expected. Perhaps Carter had been right to say this was a bad idea, and Anne even more so. But they hadn't stopped him. It was clear how badly he wanted to be out and about.

He lowered himself onto the rear-facing seat, exchanged greetings with Belinda, who was holding Rebecca, and tried to give the wide-eyed Henry a grin. But the way the child cozied up to his mother in their front-facing seat Peter figured he presented an appearance more fearsome than friendly, in spite of the newly purchased clothing and shoes he wore.

Arthur leaned in and settled the large basket Mrs. Pettigrew had provided at Peter's feet. He paused, then, raked Peter with an assessing look, and frowned. "Are you all right?"

Peter filled his chest with summer air. The raging back pain settled into the mild gnawing of an angry rodent and he replied, "I'm ready for a picnic. How about you, Henry?"

The boy nodded, eyes skimming the basket and likely looking for sweets. "Papa and I are going fishing!"

Arthur gave a laugh and settled into the driver's seat, picked up the reins and looked back at his passengers before saying, "I've a nice spot in mind. It's not far, near the road, and has the perfect blend of grass, sun, shade, and water."

"And fish!" Henry shouted.

"And fish," his father agreed. Then he signaled the horses and set them off down the road.

While Belinda engaged the baby Rebecca with a rattle, Henry's attention was snagged by the fishing poles propped against the seat, his small fingers stroking the round lengths of smooth wood. Peter watched the passing scenery and tried to keep his wound and underlying fractured shoulder blade from pressing uncomfortably against anything. The fells rose around them in every direction, craggy brown dirt and gray rock contrasting with the fresh carpet of green grass. High above, a hawk floated on outstretched wings.

After a few minutes, he returned his gaze to Belinda and found her unfocused gaze staring through his chest. "How often do you get to enjoy a family outing like this?" he asked.

She jerked. Her gaze sharpened and darted to his face, but little Rebecca began to cry and Belinda tightened her hold of the infant and patted her back.

"I startled you. I'm sorry."

Belinda switched from patting to jiggling. The baby's cries sputtered and stopped, and Peter gazed at those small, glimmering hazel eyes framed by wet, dark lashes. Ivory skin, a pink rosebud mouth, and brown curls escaping the edges of a beribboned bonnet completed the picture of infantile perfection.

"She's truly lovely," he told her mother.

Belinda looked tired, but the words brought a small smile to her lips. "Thank you. Arthur is such a proud papa. He thinks she's the most winsome baby he's ever seen."

Peter took another look. "She is. Without a doubt."

A subtle glow of pleasure suffused Belinda's face. "In answer to your question, this is our first outing of the summer, but we try to enjoy fine weather whenever possible. July tends to be our sunniest month."

"I'm grateful you included me," Peter said. "Not only is it wonderful to get out for a few hours, it's a relief to drop the pretense of another identity."

Belinda's lips thinned and her brow furrowed. "Deception is wearing, I'd imagine, even when done with good intentions."

She turned her gaze to the countryside and fell silent then, and Peter stayed quiet too. Was she referring to him, or to her father? Or perhaps her mind had turned to Emma Albright, who'd spent more than twenty years professing her innocence and Kenton's guilt. Belinda would see that as—

A flash of blue caught his attention. The water was already in sight. A few minutes later, the clarence was alongside a grassy, tree-studded area about fifty feet from the shore and approaching a particularly fine, spreading oak. Arthur slowed the rig, and as soon as it came to a stop Henry launched himself free, ran toward the lake, and began pitching pebbles.

"Make him stay back from the water," Belinda ordered.

"Henry, come away from the edge," Arthur called, heading to help Peter.

"Take care of what you need to. I'll wait," Peter told him.

Belinda handed little Rebecca down to her husband and disembarked. Walking to the base of the oak, she spread a blanket half in shade and half in dappled sunlight, and placed the baby upon it. Then she settled herself beside the infant while Arthur retrieved the food basket and set it near her. Peter relaxed and enjoyed the domestic scene, and the waters of Buttermere, clear and glorious, that stretched before him. Gentle, wind-driven waves lapped the shore.

Arthur unhitched and hobbled the horses where they could graze until it was time to leave. Then he helped Peter down.

"Sun or shade?" he asked once Peter stood beside him.

"There." Peter indicated the oak's trunk, which he could use for support if his energy faded, and with Arthur providing a strong handhold he joined Belinda and the baby on the blanket. Arthur went to the carriage, then returned with the fishing poles, a small bucket, and a bag, all of which he laid on the ground.

Henry ran back and looked up at his father, his chest puffed out. "Papa, hurry!" He looked around as if wondering at the delay. "I want a big one."

"After we eat," Arthur said in a firm tone.

Attention redirected to the picnic, Henry plopped down. His father stepped to the water, crouched and rinsed horse off his hands, then joined the rest of them on the blanket, saying, "At last. All of us together. I'm so glad you're improved, Peter, enough to have come out here."

Belinda drew Mrs. Pettigrew's basket close and sifted through the contents. After spreading several napkins on the blanket, she pulled out some paper-wrapped food, unwrapped it and arranged it atop the cloths: cheese, berries, chicken, and bread. Pickles. With a smile, she handed one napkin-wrapped bundle to Arthur, who smelled it and began peeling back the folds.

"Mmmm, gingerbread. My favorite."

Belinda cast her husband a sidelong glance. "It's Henry's favorite, too."

Henry's eyes widened. He stretched out his hand and made a wordless begging noise, in response to which Arthur moved the sweet out of his son's reach.

"Not yet. What do we do first?"

Henry folded his hands. "Pray."

"Mmm-hmm. Then what?"

Henry's mouth turned down. "I have to eat before I get a treat."

Arthur shot Peter an amused, brows-raised look. "Exactly."

Belinda withdrew corked bottles of lemonade and distributed them. Each person had a clean square of thick paper to place their food upon, and then Arthur folded his hands and bowed his head.

"Let us pray."

Peter couldn't resist watching Henry, who had the same dark hair and unruly forelock as his father. His small folded hands, his eyes squeezed tight then popping open to stare at the gingerbread, made warmth fill Peter's chest, and then an odd heaviness. He had one day hoped to have a son just like this.

After a spirited "Amen" from Henry, Arthur uncorked a lemonade and set it beside Peter's free arm. They all began to eat, and contentment seeped into Peter's bones. It had been a long while since he'd had a day so pleasant.

After the food was consumed—including sizable portions of gingerbread—Arthur, Henry, and their fishing poles adjourned to the water. Henry carried his own boy-sized pole, and Peter drew his smaller sketchpad from his pocket and began sketching father and son. Belinda packed up the remains of their repast. She'd been quiet, answering Peter's occasional questions but leaving most of the conversation to the cousins. She hadn't eaten much, and Peter recalled Arthur's worry—not only of Belinda's upset after attending the heartbreaking childbirth, but of her change of disposition since Rebecca's birth. Thin and subdued, she was unquestionably a different woman than he remembered.

"We'll have to do this again before I leave Buttermere," he said, trying to engage her in conversation.

Belinda made a humming sound but kept her gaze trained on the lake, so Peter tried again.

"Your father's invited me to finish my recuperation at Pennyton Park. Once he's back, maybe I'll move there—assuming I haven't had any new fevers."

Arthur's wife was silent, and Peter couldn't guess her feelings on the subject. Another person's feelings would affect him more, however. What if Anne hated him after he moved? And how would he avoid offending his godfather when certain questions now needed to be answered? Once within the security of Kenton's estate, he'd have no further reason to conceal his identity. He ached to tell Anne the truth and stop lying, but how would she receive the news of his long friendship with Kenton?

Belinda's eyes found Peter's. In color and shape they reminded him even more strongly of Anne, except Belinda's held a sharpness incongruous with the perfect ease of the day.

"You're still having fevers?"

"I developed a wound abscess three days ago, but Carter drained it and I felt better. We've got it well in hand," he said, hoping it was true. "The man assures me fevers are part of the healing process, and in time they will stop. For now, though, it's convenient and wise to be near him."

Belinda turned her attention back to the lake. She'd removed Rebecca's bonnet, and the baby had fallen asleep, and now she watched her husband and son fish. Peter left her to her thoughts and did the same, concentrating on his sketch. He applied the finishing marks just as Arthur pulled in his line, collected Henry's pole, and the pair headed back.

Peter considered the drawing. It was a nice one. Arthur and Henry stood side-by-side on the pebbly shore, and the tilt of Henry's head and line of his body mirrored Arthur's. Removing the page, he extended it to Belinda.

"Would you like this?"

She took the drawing, and her obvious fatigue was replaced by a look of pleasure. "This is delightful!"

"No bites," Henry called. The unhappy turn of the boy's mouth matched the dissatisfaction in his voice, and Belinda's brows bunched. Her smile went flat.

"Look, Henry," she said. She gave the sketch another glance, then tossed the drawing toward the boy, which landed at his feet.

"It's me and Papa!" The child grabbed it up, chortled, and slapped it against his chest. "Look, Papa!"

He held the drawing up, waving it wildly, and Arthur took the now crumpled drawing from his son. He studied it with a glad smile and said, "Peter, this is wonderful. May we keep it?"

Peter glanced at Belinda, whose gaze was focused on her husband. "Yes. I gave it to Belinda."

"You did?" Arthur frowned and looked at his wife. "Why did you give it to Henry, Belinda? It's creased and smeared with dirt now. We could have framed it."

Belinda shrugged and stood. She said nothing.

Arthur's mouth tightened. He folded the paper with care and tucked it inside his coat, then he looked at Peter, regret and worry shining from his eyes, and Peter suddenly remembered his cousin's comments about Belinda's mercurial moods.

He lifted his arm and offered an outstretched hand, hoping to get Arthur's mind off his problems. "I hope you saved some strength to get me on my feet."

"Don't you want to wait until after I hitch the horses?"

"I need to stand and stretch," Peter said. "Maybe Henry will show me what he's collected and stowed in his pockets." The boy had filled them to bulging with small rocks.

Arthur nodded.

As hard as Peter tried, he wasn't able to withhold a grunt of discomfort as his cousin hoisted him up. Belinda, whom he caught watching, didn't comment, and the ride back was painful and silent.

CHAPTER FIFTEEN

Anne entered the surgery back door, hung up her bonnet and scarf, and advanced into the kitchen. Mrs. Pettigrew looked up from the pot she stirred and greeted her.

"Good morning," Anne said in return. "And how is Mr. Matthews this morning?"

She'd spent the evening reassuring herself that her worries regarding yesterday's outing were excessive, but she'd been away on home visits when he returned and hadn't been able to reassure herself that he'd avoided exacerbating his injury. Since the moment she awakened she'd thought of little else.

"He's still asleep."

"Oh?" That was unusual. The last few days Peter had been awake and already breakfasted by the time she arrived. Sleeping late could mean he was healing, having less pain, or was especially tired from yesterday's excursion. It could also signal a change for the worse.

"Where's Mr. Carter? Has he seen Mr. Matthews?"

"He left right when I arrived. Said he expected to have a busy day and needed to start his visits early. He told me to let Mr. Matthews sleep and he'd check him when he returned." Mrs. Pettigrew stopped stirring and smoothed her hands over her apron. "Should I dish up his porridge?"

"Not yet. Let me take his measure first."

Anne hurried to the convalescent room to find Peter's bedcovers kicked to the foot of the bed, his face flushed, and him breathing heavy, but he slept. Unease twined through her, and it took no more than an instant of contact with his skin for her heartbeat to double its tempo. She gave his uninjured but burning hot shoulder a gentle squeeze.

"Mr. Matthews."

He didn't react, so she gave the shoulder a shake.

"*Peter.*"

He grimaced, moaned, and opened his eyes. Her relief almost made her knees buckle, as she'd been afraid he would be unresponsive.

"You have a fever."

She wasn't sure he understood. The space between his brows creased. Then his forehead smoothed and his lips curved.

"Anne. You're here."

That voice. It was raspy, like a saw against wood. He was sick. Really sick. Enough out of his head that he'd called her by her first name, too. A pitcher sat atop the nearby chest of drawers, and Anne filled the nearby cup, slipped her arm under his pillow, and lifted his head.

"Drink this," she said, putting the cup to his lips and tipping water toward his mouth.

His lips found the rim, and he drank, Anne controlling how much by tilting the cup. After several swallows, he pressed against her arm, she withdrew the cup, eased his head down, and noticed his breathing had become a little faster and more labored. The simple act of drinking had been exertion enough to make him short of breath.

"Thank you," he whispered, and his eyes fluttered closed. "You really are so sweet, taking care of me."

Anne's heart pinched. She'd found, in general, unpleasant people were disagreeable when sick; they tended to curse and want their own way even more than usual. Good-hearted people remained polite and appreciative, as Peter had been since his arrival, and that only endeared him to her further. Even four days ago, when Edwin opened Peter's infected wound, he'd joked with her afterward. This was a rare man. A fine man. And now... She filled her lungs and let the air out slow—after two weeks of care, the real challenge had arrived. The one they'd feared.

Had she played a part in this deterioration? Her throat tightened, and remorse burned like a mantle of fire across her shoulders. She'd worried yesterday's picnic would overtax him, but she hadn't told him no. Her desire that he enjoy a few hours pleasure had kept her silent. Edwin hadn't liked the idea of the outing, either, but Peter's determination had finally swayed him. They should have stayed strong, though. Just like Anne should have managed William Snow better.

Was it as bad as she feared? This high fever with altered sensorium would be a sign of pyemia, when infection advanced to the bloodstream. That was a killer. Anne would do everything she could to help him survive, but no treatment or medicine she or Edwin could provide was known to be effective. In truth, only Peter's inherent strength, and God, would determine whether he'd live.

Anne folded her hands and prayed.

Afterwards, she felt calmer. More in control. After lowering the blankets, she wet a cloth and pressed it to Peter's hot face and neck. Behind her, she heard Mrs. Pettigrew's steps and rustling skirt sweep into the room then stop before the woman murmured a distressed, "Oh, dear."

"He has a high fever," Anne said. "He'll need beef tea and puddings and soups. And when Michael arrives, he's to get a message to my mum. I'll need her to sit with him tonight."

She envied her mother that, actually. As a nurse Anne was granted considerable freedom of conduct, but there *were* limits. Given her age and unmarried status, the community would never accept Anne staying past bedtime in a home occupied by two lone, unrelated, sleeping men, no matter the circumstances. Mum's advanced age—and, as unfair as it was, her already damaged reputation—allowed her to go places and do things her daughter couldn't. People might shake their heads and whisper amongst themselves, but there'd be no more serious repercussions.

"I'll send Michael first thing," Mrs. Pettigrew said. "The poor man," she added, heading back toward the kitchen.

Hard and sharp fear filled Anne's chest like shovelfuls of gravel, weighing her down and making it a struggle to swallow. Buttermere was a small community. Discounting those at the slate mine, her patients were people she knew. She worshipped with them, had gone to school with them or their children, and considered many friends. It was as she'd discussed with Peter, how she'd suffered with Nancy. Part of nursing was grappling with emotions connected to personalizing her patients' conditions. Fear like this, though... She wasn't accustomed to this horrible, almost paralyzing fear. She didn't want to lose Peter Matthews, and that need was greater than any she'd felt for any other patient before him.

He's not yours to lose.

The thought came fast, but a refutation came just as quickly, a wave of soul-deep certainty. No matter that two weeks ago they'd been strangers, they'd forged a special and deep connection. A type of connection she'd never felt with anyone else.

Anne opened the window wide. Cold, early morning air filled the room, and she paused a moment, focused on the dew covering the hydrangea bush, and she steeled herself for the long hours and days ahead. She *would not* think about what, in the end, always occurred when someone had pyemia. She'd never seen a recovery.

The next few hours were spent trying to lower Peter's temperature. Anne applied cold cloths to his skin, fanned him, gave him water dosed with tincture of white willow, and cup after cup of beef tea. But no luck. The blistering fever didn't break.

Late in the afternoon she heard Edwin arrive. He exchanged words with Mrs. Pettigrew and a moment later appeared toting a box, which he set next to Peter's boots. "Looks like some books he ordered came," he said. Then, straightening, Edwin strode to the bed and seemed to take everything in with a sweep of his eyes.

"He's difficult to arouse but cooperative when he's awake," Anne explained. "He's blazing hot, and dry, and the fever hasn't eased at all since I got here."

Edwin shook his head and pressed his fingers to Peter's pulse. "Pyemia."

She'd known, but hearing Edwin voice the diagnosis was like a black cloud blocking the sun's last rays. Anne stifled a groan as he continued.

"We'll have a couple more days like this before the delirium begins. We're in for a rough time of it."

"Can he survive? Is it possible?"

She didn't care that her voice shook. Let Edwin think what he would; she had to know.

Edwin gave a gusty sigh, removed his spectacles, and rubbed his eyes. Very much afraid of his answer, Anne waited. Outside, she heard the sounds of someone arriving and recognized the footsteps, while Edwin shoved his eyeglasses back on and scraped back a lock of hair that had fallen over his forehead.

"Mum," Anne said as her mother stepped into the room.

"Welcome, Emma," Edwin added, his look of weariness vanishing.

"Hello," Anne's mother said to them both. "I'm sorry Mr. Matthews has taken a turn for the worse."

"I asked her to watch him tonight," Anne explained as Edwin gave her a questioning look.

He shot an assessing glance at Peter and nodded. "He'll need close watching, and more than I can give. If you want me during the night, ring the bell," Edwin instructed her mother. "That'll wake me."

"Can he recover?" Anne asked again.

"The general consensus is surviving pyemia is possible but rare. I've never had a patient live through it, and I've never known any physician or surgeon who claimed a survival. The Lancet published an account of two patients who survived, though. That's the best I can offer."

It was almost nothing, yet hope flared like a skyrocket in Anne's chest. "Two?"

"Yes. The author kept meticulous records over the entire course of his career. In *all those years*, the physician had two patients survive pyemia. One was a young boy, the other an adult man. For both, the delirium stage lasted about fourteen days."

Anne's ears buzzed. So, it was possible. Unlikely but possible.

"Were they given any different treatment?" she asked.

"No. Nothing different than every other patient." Edwin shrugged. "They just...lived. It took them several months to fully recover, though."

"Mr. Matthews was in good health when he was shot, and he's received the best possible care," Anne's mother spoke up. "He couldn't have a better surgeon or nurse. That should count for something."

Edwin ducked his head and rubbed the back of his neck. "I worried when his wound became infected, but he seemed to rebound right away. When he insisted on yesterday's outing with the Jennetts, I found his determination encouraging. He seemed healthier than this setback suggests."

"Could yesterday's activity or last week's fall have made a difference?" Anne asked. She hated the idea that her actions might have made him sicker.

"We don't know why some infected wounds heal and others spread to the blood," Carter said, seeming to read her mind, "but I'm certain nothing we did caused this. It happened *in spite* of all we did. We both warned Mr. Matthews that he should stay in bed."

Yes, they had. And Peter Matthews had made his own decision, as much as she hated any dire result that might arise from it. As much as she feared losing him.

The front door bell tinkled, and Anne went to see who had arrived. Another shock, but she quickly fought it off. Lady Kenton and her dark-haired maid, Rosella Brown, stood in the empty reception area, Miss Brown gripping the very pale viscountess's elbow.

Anne shut the treatment room door and hoped the situation could be attended quickly. "Good day, Lady Kenton. May I be of assistance?"

Instead of answering, the woman pulled her arm from Miss Brown's grip and, with a billow of green silk, sat in one of the waiting area chairs. She pulled a snowy handkerchief from her sleeve and pressed it to her eyes, appearing in some distress, and Anne felt mean that her reaction was curiosity rather than any softer feeling of concern, but on the rare occasions they had been forced to acknowledge one another, Lady Kenton's green eyes were hard as bottle glass. The viscountess didn't care to speak to her? Fine. Anne preferred talking with the blue-eyed maid, whom she knew from church services.

"Good day, Miss Albright," Miss Brown said. She gave Anne a short smile that left an impression of discomfort rather than the warmth to which Anne was more accustomed. "Lady Kenton is in need of tonic for her megrim." The maid cast an anxious look toward her employer. "I'm afraid it's quite urgent. The pain struck suddenly, after a visit with Mrs. Jennett and my lady's grandchildren. Her London physician says she's to take laudanum when this occurs."

"I'll ask Mr. Carter," Anne said. "How often does she use it?"

"Several times a month," Miss Brown replied. "It's a condition of long standing."

Lady Kenton lifted her head and glared at her maid. "Brown forgot to pack my tonic, and I've a megrim building." The maid drooped, and Lady Kenton turned her disdain on Anne. "I need to get to my bed as soon as possible. My personal physician, Dr. Avery, has a prominent London practice and is well versed with my condition. He prescribes laudanum for these attacks. Nothing else helps." Her chin jutted forward. "I expect Carter to follow Dr. Avery's direction."

Whether he would remained to be seen, but Anne couldn't wait to turn this muddle over to him. She opened the door leading into the treatment room and found herself face-to-face with Edwin and her mother.

Edwin looked past Anne into the reception area, grabbed her mother and pulled her away from the door, back into the treatment room and out of sight. Anne joined them, shutting the door behind her as Edwin turned to her mum. His hands grasped her arms, they looked at each other a moment, and then Edwin grimaced.

"It's Lady Kenton, Emma," he said, his voice deep and soft. Anne's mother's lips parted and her eyes widened as he added, "There's no need for you to involve yourself. Stay with Mr. Matthews. Anne and I will take care of this."

The two stared into each other's faces, and Edwin's thumbs rubbed Anne's mother's upper arms. Anne saw her mum's face go pink, then she pulled free of Edwin's steadying grip and hurried back to the convalescent room.

Anne gave Edwin an account of her conversation with Lady Kenton and Rosella Brown. "Did you know she regularly suffers from headaches? Strong ones?"

"No. I've never treated Lady Kenton for anything."

"Shall I fetch a bottle of laudanum?"

"I suppose so," Edwin said. "It sounds like the lady knows what she needs."

Anne collected the laudanum and a glass of water, and when she returned to the reception area Lady Kenton stood explaining her condition to Edwin, eyes closed and fingers pressed against her temples. Miss Brown stepped forward. Anne uncorked the bottle and poured a dose into the water, and the maid took it straight to her employer, who grabbed the glass and drank it down.

"Send for me if the laudanum doesn't give you relief," Edwin said when she was done.

"Very well," Lady Kenton replied.

"I'll stop by tomorrow and speak to Lord Kenton."

"There's no need. My husband is still in Berkshire, engaged with equine matters. I'll be fine now that I have my medicine." Lady Kenton gave Miss Brown a pointed look and raised her brows, and the maid lifted the bottle, verifying her possession.

"All right," Edwin said. "If you're sure."

"I'm very sure. Good day." The viscountess's green silk swirled, she snapped out her maid's name, and a moment later the pair was gone. Without a single word of thanks.

Edwin moved to the window. "There's a driver waiting." He gave a chuckle and echoed Anne's own thoughts. "Her gratitude overwhelms me."

Anne couldn't quite keep the scorn from her voice. "She's a viscountess. Surely you know what an honor it is to care for her. What other reward could we possibly want?"

Edwin glanced at her then said, "Why don't we all have dinner together before you leave? You, me and your mother."

"Shouldn't you check with Mrs. Pettigrew before issuing such rash invitations?"

Edwin looked amused. "She may have already said there was plenty."

"I don't want him to die."

The words had come out of nowhere and filled the space between them. Stricken, Anne stared at Edwin, whose smile had dropped.

"I know," he said. Then he patted her shoulder and headed toward the kitchen.

Anne returned to Peter's bedside, where nothing had changed. He was no worse, but that wasn't much to hang on to. That reality must have shown on her face, because Anne's mother wrapped an arm around her shoulders and held her tight.

~

Pain and heat seared Peter's body, turned his blood to pulsing, boiling lava. His head throbbed so hard that it hurt to open his eyes. Thank God for Anne. Her presence calmed and fortified him, and he soaked it up. Whenever she placed a cold pad across his forehead, it didn't lessen the pain, but it did confer a bit of relief, a stark pleasure in the midst of so much misery. A pinpoint oasis upon his desert of a body.

He followed her commands, swallowing whatever she spooned into his mouth. Tried not to worry about how much sicker he seemed to be. Anne and Carter both tended him, and sometimes by lamplight or moonlight, Anne's mother.

Sleep, at first an escape, became more wearing than restorative. Once, he woke and found his fiancée standing over him.

"Louisa?" He reached out, tried to catch a fold of her skirt, but the cool, gossamer fabric slipped through his fingers like the silkiest shadow.

She seemed different in ways he couldn't define. Not her appearance: Louisa's loveliness and confidence hadn't altered. If anything, her beauty shone more luminous than ever. Her eyes still gleamed with intelligence, and the patient smile that put everyone from pauper to prince at ease curved her rosy lips. So, why didn't her perfection rouse the same admiration and satisfaction and pride he'd always felt in her presence? Could *he* be the one changed? Because that perfect harmony was gone.

He'd rather have Anne beside him. There was no denying it. He tried to ignore the guilt pressing against his chest, tried to offer Louisa a reassuring word, but his mouth wouldn't move. When she finally slipped away, his reaction was as much a sense of liberation as loss.

Days wheeled by. After a time, he got worse. He wanted to wake up and couldn't. Not completely. Thank God he still felt Anne there. He could discern her touch; he knew when she was there and not someone else. And then the pall lifted, except he was in Appleseed Lake, swimming from the bottom to the surface and running out of air. How had he gotten in the lake? And what were Anne and Carter doing at Treewick Hall? He could barely hear their voices through the water. He shouldn't have gone so deep.

Fear twisted his belly. He'd gone too deep.

His ears ached. Too deep. Too much pressure.

He strained for the surface as some of their words drifted down. Pyemia. Suppurative fever. Acute stage. Delirium. Mostly the words were gibberish, mere meaningless sounds; they circled inside his brain, whirled in unison with the godawful pounding. Occasionally he was aware, though. The pain. The heat. Her hands. Liquid in his mouth. He swallowed. Felt her approval. So he tried, as hard as he could, to swim up close enough to grab a breath of air and swallow again.

His stomach became a black, bottomless pit. His flesh shriveled; his organs turned to bricks. Anne's voice remained his one comfort, nourished his last shred of will. He held on to her presence and trusted she'd guide him to the surface. And then, for one moment, she did. In a moment of clear-headedness, he found her beside him. One long, fiery strand of hair had escaped its pin. That brilliant lock swayed, glinted in the light. He reached for it, but his arm was too heavy.

"Peter?"

She looked tired.

Oh. He remembered.

"I…I'm…sick."

What was wrong with his mouth? He tried to wet it with his tongue, but that wasn't working right either. Her eyes filled, and Anne looked at the ceiling. She blinked, again and again. Looked down, closed her eyes. Nodded.

Oh. No.

"Not…dying," he managed. Didn't she know that? She should. He didn't think she'd let him die, even if God decreed it.

She laughed—or sobbed. He wasn't sure which. Then she gave him a quivery smile. Sniffed. Nodded again. This time with strength and purpose. Her palm stroked the hair from his forehead, and…it felt nice, but cold?

Chills whisked over his flesh. He shuddered and fell back into the dark waters of Appleseed Lake.

CHAPTER SIXTEEN

Arthur's voice droned on, prodding him from sleep.

"Ungh. Be *quiet,*" Peter begged.

"Praise God!"

"What…?" His cousin's voice had held such joy that it brought Peter fully awake. Arthur didn't get excited; it took a significant occurrence to sway his unruffled demeanor. He blinked gritty eyes, bringing his cousin into focus. Even without knowing the cause of the gladness, Peter felt his chest fill with happiness at that broad smile.

"I can tell from your voice you've returned to your senses. You've been delirious."

A hazy recollection of disjointed images flashed through Peter's mind, along with the more recent and lucid memory of waking with hair, skin, and sheets soaking wet, and Anne's voice saying, excited as a child's on Christmas morning, "Your fever's broken." It seemed cause for celebration, but he'd fallen asleep.

"I feel better," he murmured. He lifted his hand to his jaw and found a fuller beard. For a moment he froze with surprise, then his arm began to ache and tremble. He let it fall to his chest, saying, "I'm weak as an infant. How long…?"

"A fortnight."

Fourteen days! That surprised him more than finding his overlong whiskers had filled out into a beard. "I've been out of my head for two weeks?" He struggled to work out the passage of time, which had been...about thirty-five days since he'd been shot. Astonishing. A quick look above showed the spider's web had doubled in size.

"Carter called it a medical crisis." His cousin shoved his hand through his hair, obviously relieved. "We didn't know if you'd live."

Peter looked down at his body, considered how it felt. Warm in a comfortable way. Sore and weak. Alert and...*hungry*. Relief and gladness built in his chest and quivered there, a tension similar to the burgeoning pressure that formed prior to tears. A dry-eyed version of extreme emotion. He cleared his throat and offered, "I believe I've survived."

"You're the only person I know who'd interrupt my prayer to tell me to be quiet. Given that you seem your overbearing self, I'd say you're correct." Arthur's voice held frothy lightness, but his eyes sparkled with unshed tears.

"I have the impression you've been here a lot?"

"Every day. But don't worry, your secret's still safe. Carter and Miss Albright believe you and I became friends during my visits when we played cards and chess. Add to that my pastoral duties, and no one has reason to question why I'd spend so much time by your side."

"I wasn't worried," Peter said. He'd actually forgotten about the charade completely. "I think I remember Anne's mother...?"

"She spelled Carter during the nights. And Miss Albright's been here from early morning to late evening every day."

So, Anne had gotten him through the suppurative fever. Others helped, but it was Anne's care—and caring—that had sustained him. Her touch and voice had poked like little miracles through the impenetrable miasma of fever; her presence kept at bay the suffocating panic and helplessness, as acute as the day he battled Death in the river that took his parents and Louisa. This time, Anne had been with him and he'd won. He was *alive*.

His cousin stood and walked to the table by the window. Outside, the hydrangea seemed more blue blossom than green foliage. Arthur picked up a stack of envelopes and sifted through them, reading each in turn.

"You've letters. One's from Owen Weaver. The others are from George Lawton and Henry Nickerson." He tapped the edges against his open palm. "Isn't Nickerson your man of business?"

Peter let his dazzling happiness fade to a rosy glow. "He is. Lawton is the engineer I hired to evaluate Bellow Hill." He hoped the letter meant Lawton had a solution. "They're all addressed to Matthews?"

"Yes," Arthur confirmed.

"Good. That means Weaver talked to him. Hand Weaver's over, will you?"

Arthur gave him one, Peter opened it and managed to skim through the missive before the page grew too heavy. He let his arm drop, saying, "In chasing the man who tried to kill me, he's ruled out most of the more likely miners—those speaking out against me—but now he's investigating the angriest and most vocal of the lot. And then there's Hardesty. I hate suspecting him, but he and this angry miner seem the prime suspects. Not that Hardesty would do it himself. He'd definitely hire someone to do the dirty work." He extended the letter, which Arthur took and put back inside its envelope. Then Peter said, "I'll read the others after I eat. They'll make better sense once my brain's been fed."

Arthur nodded and placed the envelopes back on the table.

"Speaking of food, could you fetch Anne?" Peter asked. "Or Mrs. Pettigrew? Tell them I'd like to eat."

Arthur settled his smooth-domed hat on his head and smiled, clearly thrilled that all was back to normal. "I'm pleased to be able to return to my duties for the church. I'll find one of the ladies on my way out." He paused in the doorway. "And thank you for the good night's sleep I'm going to have tonight."

As his cousin left, Peter waited and listened. His attentiveness was rewarded when he heard Anne's footsteps approaching, and how they hurried. He had memorized the cadence of her walk, he realized.

She rushed in, face beaming, and felt his forehead. When she stepped back and sank onto the chair, her shining eyes and grinning mouth made his throat tighten. She giggled—giggled!—and pressed her hand to her chest.

"You're going to be fine!"

Those words erupted, quick and breathy, like she'd just finished a foot race, and the sight of her—happy and laughing because of *him*—felt a lot like reaching Grossglockner's summit. Peter basked in the pleasure.

"I feared you wouldn't live. So many don't."

"My spirit knew better than to pass over," Peter offered. "My ghost could never have borne your wrath."

Anne laughed. "I didn't realize ghosts would find me fearsome."

"Well, I'm certain mine would. Your displeasure would have made my poor specter miserable. You've saved yourself all manner of blood-curdling wails."

She eyed him, and the shudder she gave was big. "I imagine you'd be a right grumpy ghost."

"I'll be a crotchety patient if I don't get food in my belly."

Anne stood. "Aren't I fortunate then, since Mrs. Pettigrew is warming something now. She won't be long. Let's get you ready."

Even with help, sitting up and getting pillows stuffed around and behind him was exhausting.

"Maybe soup would be best—in a mug," he added. He thought he could manage drinking, but eating with a utensil would require a steadier hand than he possessed. Anne had spoon-fed him on several occasions, but he didn't want her doing that now.

His empty stomach *hurt* by the time Mrs. Pettigrew arrived, indeed bringing soup. Anne returned to the cushioned chair while Peter drank the potage of chicken, noodles, peas and carrots. It was the best—the absolute *best*—he'd ever had, and Anne got him another cup without his asking. He began falling asleep before he'd finished. She plucked the cup from his hand, and he slid down into the warm bedcovers as he said, "You think I'll recover completely now?"

"Yes," she said, smiling again. "But it could take two months before you're well enough to leave Buttermere on your horse."

Two months? A long time to be weak and at the mercy of his

assailant. Not that he'd had any inkling of the man, which meant this was truly a safe hideaway after all.

"What can I do to hasten my recovery?"

"Eat. Sleep."

He could do that. When he woke he would read his other letters, too. For now he would enjoy his full stomach and the knowledge that he was alive and on his way to being well.

Peter closed his eyes. Anne's petticoats rustled as she left, and from the direction of the kitchen Mrs. Pettigrew began to sing another of those sea shanties he sometimes heard from her. Anne's voice joined Mrs. Pettigrew's for the final chorus, harmonizing nicely, and Peter barked out a laugh. She had never done that before. Could she be as happy as he was?

The intensity of his banked happiness grew, spread, and filled him. Smiling, he drifted toward sleep…until a sudden thought jolted him awake and replaced his contentment with apprehension.

While he'd been insensible, had Anne accepted Snow or Carter's proposal?

~

Anne always enjoyed the scenery on her walks home. The days were so long right now, she had the benefit of lovely landscapes, even though the lake lay south and out of sight of the cottage she and Mum shared. The fells: Robinson, Grasmoor, and High Stile surrounded her, Herdwick sheep and the occasional deer wandering freely on the grassy, heather-strewn slopes. The spring bluebells had died off, but this month dog roses and butterflies abounded, and her favorite patch of meadowsweet filled the air with fragrance when she strolled past. It was a good time of year for many of the local medicinal plants she collected; she should take a day for collecting.

A bunny darted from a roadside shrub, making her pause and remember one of Peter's sketches of a rabbit hidden in a cluster of flowers. She recalled how he'd looked today, his fever gone, smiling and happy again. Free of the last two weeks' worry, she felt light enough to float.

She'd just turned up the bungalow path when the sound of an approaching carriage made her stop. She turned, and Belinda Jennett pulled up a horse and chaise easily recognizable as belonging to Lord Kenton.

"Get in," Belinda cried. "Dr. Carter isn't home, and I need someone."

Anne's stomach dropped. "What's happened?"

"It's my mother. She fell and hit her head. It won't stop bleeding. The cut needs to be stitched."

Lady Kenton? Anne didn't want to go with Belinda to attend, but if Edwin wasn't available... They would never ask her mother, which just left her. Except, Anne had never been inside Pennyton Park. She wasn't even sure she could force her feet across the threshold.

"Where is she?" she asked.

"At the parsonage."

Oh. That explained Belinda fetching Anne with a Pennyton Park horse and carriage: Lady Kenton must have driven herself to her daughter's house. If Lady Kenton had been at her own home, a servant would have been dispatched to fetch Edwin.

"Please, hurry," Belinda said. "My husband's not at home. I left my children with my mother, and she's distraught."

Her half-sister's voice held sharp condemnation, as if it would be Anne's fault if something horrible happened. There was nothing else to do but go. "Just a moment. I'll get my kit."

Anne proceeded into the house she shared with her mother and grabbed her medical bag. She kept the kit, in appearance similar to a single saddlebag, ready with a variety of medical supplies for use at any time.

The aroma and warmth of baking bread filled the cottage, and her mother appeared in the kitchen doorway, obviously surprised by Anne's actions. "Are you leaving?"

"Lady Kenton needs assistance, and Edwin's not available. She's at the parsonage." Anne passed her medical kit's wide strap over her left shoulder and head and positioned it across her torso so that the bag rested on her hip. Mum walked into the parlor and looked out the open front door. Her brow furrowed and her mouth went flat. Then her chin rose.

"I'm sorry you have to go."

"I'll be fine."

Anne kissed her mother's cheek and trotted out to the chaise. She climbed in, and Belinda cracked the whip. Then the horse took off.

The parsonage sat on the outskirts of Buttermere, a couple hundred yards down the road from St. James Church. Anne didn't know if Belinda were brave or harebrained to drive so fast, but she didn't object to the speed and roughness of the ride. She held tight to the seat rail instead, kept her eyes straight ahead, and prayed she wouldn't end up in a ditch.

"Did you see her fall?" she asked as they rode. "Did she lose consciousness when she hit her head?" If she had, there might be a more complicated injury than a head laceration.

"She's fine," Belinda said with a quick glance. "The cut's just bleeding a lot."

Her half-sister's matter-of-fact words belied the recklessness of her driving. But then, she'd said she was concerned for her children. The conveyance flew past the livery stable-yard and Andrew Snow, outside in the paddock, turned his head as it passed.

What he must think of her, Anne realized. She'd been absorbed in caring for Peter and barely given his proposal a thought, and it had now been over a month. How could she have ignored him for so long? He was still waiting for her answer, and he'd bothered her again not once; shame on her. Stricken, she looked back and saw him peering through the dust stirred by the racing horse and carriage, and Anne wondered which he'd consider more astonishing—their breakneck speed, Belinda's lack of a bonnet, or seeing Belinda and Anne together.

She planted her feet and held on with both hands as they turned onto the parsonage property. As soon as the chaise stopped, she jumped down. There was work to be done.

"Follow me," Belinda said. She didn't spare Anne a glance but sprinted for the front door.

Anne entered to the sound of crying children. The toddler appeared uninjured but had smears of blood on his fingers, face, and shirt. He stood in the parlor with one hand on the edge of his sister's cradle, tears streaming down his cheeks. The bright red infant looked furious, her mouth open, her body quivering from the force of her screams.

Belinda scooped up the baby, knelt and hugged the little boy close: Henry, Anne recalled. And Rebecca. She turned her attention to Lady Kenton, who sat in a rocker and apparently hadn't done much to try and stem her bleeding. Blood trickled down the side of her face and saturated a portion of her bodice, and she held a blood-soaked pad in her lap. Blood smeared the rocker arms, her dress, and soaked the right side of her head. She would have a devil of a time cleaning it from her hair. Or, rather, her lady's maid would. Red footprints—adult and toddler—marked the wood floor and rug.

"What're *you* doing here?" Lady Kenton called out, wrinkling her nose as if Anne toted offal. She batted her hand dismissively in the air.

Sluggish, somewhat slurred speech, Anne noted. Exaggerated, sloppy movements. Slow-blinking, glazed eyes with pupils too small for the subdued light. None were normal. Palsy could explain this—the woman's affected speech and coordination—and could have caused the fall, too.

"Dr. Carter isn't available," Anne said. She set her kit on the pedestal side table and fished out a compress. Scalp lacerations were often vigorous bleeders, and this one was large, half a finger-length. She pressed the compress to the laceration, but Lady Kenton drew her head away and scowled.

"I don't want you here."

That makes two of us, but I think you need me, Anne didn't say.

"I'll be quick," she offered instead. And this time, when she applied the compress, Anne kept Lady Kenton from moving away by supporting the back of her head.

A bloody hand wrapped around Anne's sleeve. "Ow!"

Anne made her voice stern. "I need to hold pressure on this until the bleeding stops."

Lady Kenton fixed her with a glare. Those eyes, they held such disapproval and dislike. They always had, from Anne's earliest memories. But gradually the clutching fingers loosened and Lady Kenton's hand dropped to her lap.

"Tell me how you happened to fall," Anne prompted.

For a long moment, Lady Kenton's face went slack. Anne was about to repeat the question when she finally answered. "I tripped over Henry's toy."

No stroke, then. The viscountess's face, mouth, and arms appeared to be moving naturally, and Anne would expect some debility if Lady Kenton had experienced one. She leaned closer, ignoring the smell of coppery blood and sweet violet cologne and sought some other clue to the woman's slurred words.

There. Something floated on Lady Kenton's breath rather than emanated from her skin. Anne caught the unmistakable scents of alcohol, clove, and cinnamon, which along with opium were the common ingredients of laudanum like she and Edwin had given the woman earlier. 'Twas likely Lady Kenton had ingested too much of what they'd prescribed. Not a palsy stroke after all.

"Where's Carter?" the viscountess rambled. "I don't want you."

"Mr. Carter may be several hours," Anne said, lifting the compress. The wound had stopped bleeding. "You may wait if you prefer, but I can suture this and be gone in fifteen minutes."

Belinda stood nearby, bouncing the gasping, hiccoughing baby. Henry clutched his mother's skirt, thumb secured in his mouth. "Let her take care of it, Mother. You've upset the children and made a mess of the house. I want things back to normal."

Surprise rippled through Anne. Belinda's commanding, chastising tone reversed the natural order of power of mother over daughter. While Anne had no idea of the level of affection these two shared, they'd always presented a united front before. Belinda sat with her parents at church services, and over the years they'd shown equal amounts of disdain for Anne and Emma Albright each.

Lady Kenton's head wobbled as she turned away. "Oh, get on with it."

"I'd like to wash my hands first, Mrs. Jennett," Anne said. "Then I'll need a basin, and wine to cleanse the wound, if you've got some."

"Of course. This way."

With a few words to Henry, Belinda detached his fingers from her skirt and left the parlor. Anne followed, through a spotless kitchen and into the attached scullery. There, Anne went to the large slate sink. She paused, considering her bloody hands.

"Let me." Belinda, still holding Rebecca with her left arm, reached past Anne to grasp the pump handle. Tight-mouthed, she pumped until a gush of water spewed from the spout.

Anne picked up the cake of lye soap and began to wash, conscious of the woman beside her. She didn't think they'd ever been this physically close. Rebecca looked like a drooling cherub, waving her arms in her mother's grip, and Anne had the sudden urge to pluck her from Belinda, hug her solid, damp warmth and smell her sweet, talcumy baby scent. To know her niece.

Belinda suddenly shifted the infant onto her shoulder and tugged the blanket up, concealing Rebecca's head. The movement unexpectedly cut to Anne's very core, slicing through the scarred gall walling off the pain of Anne's parentage, and her half-sister's gaze was no less sharp.

Hurt oozed into Anne's chest. She couldn't breathe. This must be how young Tim Elmore felt when he couldn't get air into his lungs. She steeled herself against the suffocating squeeze, and suddenly anger erupted like a fountain of molten rock. Air rushed back into her lungs and her hands stilled. Why, for so many years, had she acted such a coward, stuffing her anger—and yes, her shame—deep inside? Dissembling was exhausting. She was *sick* of the pretense. Of feigning she and Belinda were no more than acquaintances, acquaintances who disliked each other at that. They were *sisters,* for God's sake, and they didn't even use each other's Christian names. They'd never, face-to-face, acknowledged their relation.

What was the point of all this lifelong pretending? Mum was the strongest woman Anne knew, and perfectly capable of deciding what was best for herself. So could Anne. She'd liked how it felt when she'd been honest with Peter about her history: open, unashamed, fully herself.

Belinda pumped out another stream of water, and it splashed over Anne's waiting hands. Then Belinda offered a towel. Anne's hands moved, accepting the cloth. A distant part of her noticed her hands were trembling. Their gazes collided, and Anne looked into eyes that were twins to her own.

"Belinda," she began, and Belinda started, her eyes wide, and she stepped back. "I'm finished pretending you're no more than the rector's wife. I'm *always* aware we're sisters, and I'll no longer be acting otherwise."

Rebecca made a few unhappy noises. Eyes locked on Anne, Belinda jounced the baby.

"Are we?" she asked.

How can you look in my eyes and doubt it?

But perhaps she did. Somehow, Anne had always believed Kenton's family knew the truth, but maybe, of everyone, they were the most likely to deny her parentage. It didn't change Anne's decision, but this wasn't the time to debate familial connections.

"Your mother has used a lot of laudanum today. She's stupefied."

Belinda's eyes squeezed shut. She continued to jounce her now quiet baby.

"Belinda!" Her sister's eyes shot open, and suddenly Anne knew Belinda carried her own secrets. Anne's anger streamed away, leaving nothing but compassion. "Does your mother have an unhealthy fondness for laudanum?"

There were no tears, no denials. Just a tiny line between Belinda's brows, and a sharp, affirmative nod. "She's obsessed, as if an evil spirit controls her."

It was Anne's turn to be shocked. Not by the admission, but at Belinda's tone and demeanor, both devoid of regret or sorrow. Perhaps this came from Lady Kenton's habit being a longstanding one.

"I'll let Mr. Carter know," she said. "He may be able to help."

Belinda made no response, so Anne forced her mind back to the job at hand. The two of them returned to the parlor and found Lady Kenton somnolent, hands folded in her lap. Belinda returned the baby to her cradle; Henry sat on the rug and played with an assortment of wooden animals. Anne roused Lady Kenton and explained what she'd be doing. The viscountess gave a slight nod of acknowledgment but kept her eyes closed and her head turned away, which gave Anne better access to the gash.

Belinda stood nearby watching. Quiet and calm descended.

Anne proceeded: washing the wound, fishing a silk ligature from her bag, threading the silk through the needle and closing the laceration. With the first pierce of the needle, Lady Kenton's body stiffened. She didn't move, though, and Anne continued suturing. A few minutes later Anne knotted the ligature.

"Have you any other injuries, Lady Kenton?"

"No." The lady put her rocker in motion. Her lids fluttered open, but she kept her gaze on one of several pastoral paintings. Never on Anne.

"Very well." Anne packed away her supplies, passed the medical bag's strap over her head, and settled it on her hip. "I'll walk home."

Belinda showed her out.

Anne passed through the archway, and without a good-bye or a word of thanks, the door shut.

She strode away from the parsonage, not caring she had a longer walk home than usual. There was plenty of time yet before the summer sun set, and the walk would do her good, give her an opportunity to rethink all that had occurred in the Jennett home and settle her tumbled emotions. She'd tell Edwin about Lady Kenton's fall and laudanum habit tomorrow, but telling her mum what had passed between Belinda and herself couldn't wait.

When the livery stable-yard appeared, she knew telling Andrew her decision couldn't wait, either. She'd already put him off far, far too long.

She found him in the stable, feeding the horses. He stopped when he saw her and waited as she advanced into the shadowy interior full of the warm scents of horse, leather, and hay, the sound of contented, chewing equines its own sort of music. Without a greeting, his gaze swept down her, pausing on the bloodied spots.

"Everything all right?" he asked. Once she nodded he said, "So you've remembered me, have you?" She caught the sharp gleam of anger and hurt before he turned his head away, and shame curled in her belly like a beaten dog.

"Andrew, I'm sorry I've made you wait so long for my answer. I had to be certain, and I *wasn't* certain what the right decision was. Then Mr. Matthews became very ill, and everything but nursing him went out of my head."

He looked at her. She could see that he expected her refusal, yet he waited. He was making her say it, not making it easy. But perhaps that was only fair.

She took a deep breath and prayed that deep down he'd be relieved. "You're such a dear friend, and I know we'd be comfortable together, but...when I marry, I want to feel more for my husband than love for a friend." Like Peter made her feel. Not that she'd ever tell Andrew that. She didn't want to hurt him; she just wanted them both to be happy.

"Is it partly what my dad said? Or because he's too fond of the drink?"

She hesitated. If she were honest, what Mr. Snow had said the last time she saw him mattered. It wasn't only her feeling for Peter that had clinched her decision. But the decision would surely have been the same regardless.

"That's not the reason, but I know your dad is why you're always so careful with *your* reputation. You don't like family gossip, and you strive to live an exemplary life. One beyond reproach. You've earned your reputation as an honest, warm-hearted man—a *good* man." She gripped his forearm. "You always say my illegitimacy and my mother's notoriety don't matter, but I think in time you'd find them a curse."

Andrew's eyes squeezed shut, and his head drooped. His silence seemed to confirm the truth of her statement, which she'd always suspected. But she didn't hold it against him. She gave his arm a squeeze then released it.

"Please forgive me," she begged. "This is for the best."

After a time his head lifted. He took a deep breath and gave a solemn nod. Anne rocked up onto her toes, kissed his cheek, and then hurried away.

Down the road, the tightness in her belly eased. She'd done the right thing. Someday, she hoped, he'd realize that and be glad.

CHAPTER SEVENTEEN

She arrived home well before dark. The moment she entered, her mother set aside her mending and stood.

Anne removed her bonnet, hanging it and her medical bag on a peg near the door. "Something still smells good."

"I hope you're ready to eat. I waited for you."

The high emotion she'd experienced, first with Peter, then Belinda, Lady Kenton, and finally Andrew, seemed to have left a ravenous hunger in Anne. "Just let me change first." She held up her blood smeared sleeve.

Her mother grimaced. "Perhaps we can add cuffs to cover the stain." She shrugged and shook her head. "Hurry. I'm anxious to hear how it went."

By the time Anne got to the kitchen, her mother had bread and steaming bowls of soup on the table, while behind her Phoebe strolled in, sat in front of the stove and blinked drowsy green feline eyes at them. Pure white paws and chest contrasted with the black of her coat. White whiskers sprouted from a white muzzle that extended in a stripe up the cat's forehead. Phoebe's pink nose lifted and quivered as she drank in the kitchen smells.

Anne sat, grabbed a waiting glass of water and downed it, then reached for a slice of bread and scooped butter from the crock. Where to start? So much had happened.

"Mr. Matthews's fever broke. He's clearheaded, eating and drinking. He won't need close watching anymore."

Mum had been refilling Anne's glass from the pitcher and quickly set it down. She gasped, and her lips spread in a huge smile. "He's bested the pyemia?" They clasped hands. "That's wonderful! Edwin must be happy as a dog with two tails."

Anne chuckled. "He proclaimed Mr. Matthews an official miracle and says he expects no further crises. Quite the opposite, he expects Mr. Matthews to have an uncomplicated recovery from here out."

"I'm glad, and I know you're ecstatic. He's become a friend, hasn't he?"

"He's made me rethink my life," Anne admitted. At her mother's look of surprise, she folded her hands and pressed them to her chest, which suddenly didn't hold quite enough air. She hoped Mum would understand why she'd refused Andrew Snow; her mother had encouraged her to marry him, wanting her daughter happily settled with a family of her own. But marriage to Andrew wouldn't dispel all that made her different, as Mum thought it would. Marriage certainly hadn't worked for her half-sister. Belinda had never been fully accepted into the community.

"I'm not marrying Andrew, Mum. I told him today."

Her mother's face squeezed into an expression of disappointment. Then she blinked, her eyes widened, and Anne saw puzzlement replace the dismay. "You aren't refusing him because you've formed an attachment to Mr. Matthews, are you?"

Anne straightened. Her decision hadn't been made lightly. "Mr. Matthews is an attractive and interesting man, and I admire him. He's made me realize my feelings for Andrew are those of a sister for a brother—and I want more."

Her mother's shoulders sagged. She had always stressed that with Andrew Anne would be marrying a friend, and that in time such a union would become a deeply loving one, but sisterly feelings were clearly different. Anne wished Mum hadn't sounded so appalled at the idea Anne might be attracted to Peter. Was it because he was a patient, making such a situation fodder for gossip? Because he was here for a short time and would be eventually leaving? Or simply because Mum had always favored the steadiness of Andrew?

"You know I'm disappointed," her mother said. "Was he upset?"

Anne moistened her lips. Her mum might be gauging whether Anne could change her mind once Peter was gone and his influence removed, and she didn't want Mum holding onto an impossible hope. "He wasn't surprised, and he didn't try to convince me."

"Oh."

Anne began to eat. Finally, her mother picked up her spoon. The two of them ate in silence for a time, then her mother broke the silence.

"What was wrong with Lady Kenton?"

"She had a scalp laceration. I sutured it."

Mum nodded. "And how did it go with them?"

Anne hesitated. She took a little salt from the cellar and scattered it over her soup. Even after all these years, her mum had a volatile temper when presented with any injustice perpetrated by a Kenton.

"Were they discourteous?"

Anne glanced up and saw the intensity of her mother's gaze. "Something in me snapped. I told Belinda I'm finished pretending we aren't connected."

Her mother covered the lower part of her face with her hands. After a moment her hands dropped and she shook her head. "You had quite the day, didn't you?" She straightened and leaned back. "No member of that family will ever acknowledge you in public. Stirring the pot will only make the situation worse."

"I didn't plan to challenge her," Anne admitted, "but I'm glad I did."

"Good," Mum said with a satisfied tone. "How did Belinda react?"

"She didn't. I immediately turned the topic to her mother. Lady Kenton was stupefied with laudanum." Her mother gasped, but Anne continued, "It was the reason for her fall. Belinda admitted her mother has a laudanum habit. Called her 'obsessed.'"

Mum shuddered. "Lady Kenton has spent a lifetime putting on a proud face while living with *him*."

Anne nodded slowly, but her thoughts weren't on Lord and Lady Kenton. They were on her mum. "We see them—*him*—every summer. I've never understood, not really, why Grandfather stayed in Buttermere. Or you. He was the accountant for Dale Head Mine. He could have found a position elsewhere and moved the family." She'd asked before but never pressed for answers because her mother always seemed to take Anne's questions as criticism or even accusation. It was time to get past that defensiveness, for Anne to know everything, and for her mother to know for certain that Anne held her blameless.

"Mother was the midwife," Mum said. "It would have been next to impossible finding a town that needed both a man of business and a midwife."

"They must have wanted very desperately to leave."

"Of course they did. After Father stormed over to Pennyton Park and confronted Kenton—who accused me of lying?"

"Grandfather couldn't have believed that!" Honesty was never compromised. Anne had been raised on that precept, and she knew her mother had been as well.

"He and Mother didn't, but others did." Mum folded her hands and pressed them to her chest, much as Anne often did. "I should have accused Kenton immediately. It was my waiting until I realized I was pregnant that put doubt in everyone's mind."

Anne shook her head. "Why didn't you at least tell Nan right away? I'm not criticizing you, I just want to understand." Her mother and grandmother had been close.

Her mother's hands dropped, and she took a deep breath. "I was shocked and confused. Ashamed. The way Kenton talked after he violated me, as if I'd deliberately enticed him, made me think I *was* to blame. I thought I hadn't tried hard enough to get away."

"Oh, Mum, no."

Her mother's gaze, clear and direct, didn't waver. "He was strong, and it happened fast. When I tried to push him off, he *laughed*. Later, I thought, why would he laugh? He either enjoyed hurting me, which would make him a monster, or he thought we were both enjoying ourselves."

"His mind is disturbed, that's how." She should have dragged all this from her mum years ago. To think she'd ever cast doubt or blame on herself!

"I didn't know what to do. I wanted to forget it happened. A rich, powerful aristocrat, one everyone in the community felt indebted to... He'd built the school and paid the schoolmaster's salary!" Anne's mother's hands lifted in a helpless gesture. "I thought it *must* have been at least partly my fault, because how could such a generous man do something so heinous? I was so ashamed. Finally, when I realized I was carrying you, I had to tell."

Mum shook her head, sighed, then continued. "Do you know, when Father confronted him, at first Kenton urged him to be kind. He explained my claim of rape was merely an attempt to save my reputation." She gave a dry, humorless laugh. "He said no one needed to know I'd encouraged our coupling. Everything he told Father played into my own naive doubts. Eventually, it was Mother who settled my mind. She made me realize Kenton had completely overwhelmed me. That I should trust I'd done nothing to entice him, and that some men see any act as encouragement. Especially entitled men.

"I wanted to leave, but I wasn't quite ready to strike out on my own as a midwife. With a new baby and without family support I'd have been doomed. I begged to go stay with Cousin Althea, but the idea horrified Father. If you could have seen him when he said, 'Albrights don't run away, and we take care of our own.' He was fierce. Always so proud and stubborn.

"It wasn't long before my pregnancy became the local scandal, but Mother and Father ignored it with the help of their friends. I tried to. What else was there to do after my accusation was ignored? Kenton denied the rape and never explained. I guess such men never must. Eventually the theory emerged that I seduced him and claimed rape to save my reputation, just as Kenton suggested. And so I was the one who bore the shame. I was the flirtatious harlot."

"Grandfather and Nan didn't ever believe that, did they?"

"No. I couldn't have borne it if they had. I hated that they were pitied by the ones who did believe."

"I've been pitied as well," Anne said. "Or watched for signs of damaged character. Viscount Kenton will have a lot to answer for when he's called to Judgement."

Her mother's face changed from surprise, to pain, to puzzlement. "'Signs of damaged character'? I know you've had to bear the stigma of being Kenton's illegitimate child," Mum said, "but your morals have never been questioned. Have they?"

Anne took a deep breath, not wanting to hurt her mother but also wanting her to know the truth. "There've been many days patients watch and take my measure, and I see the questions in their eyes. Those who believe Kenton look to see if I give any hint of licentiousness. Those who believe you watch for dishonesty, duplicity, and cruelty. There's no winning, as I'm the product of sin from one hand or the other."

Her mother's mouth opened with a soft gasp. "You started to say something like this when you were younger but stopped. Was it because you knew it hurt me?" She shook her head and swallowed, and her eyes glistened with unshed tears. "I'm sorry, so sorry for not realizing. After your Nan and Grandfather died, I *should* have moved us away. Except by then I was the midwife and I'd adapted." Her nose wrinkled, and her eyes went hard. "Although I've always hated facing Kenton each summer and never stopped wishing he'd somehow get a comeuppance."

Anne wished the same. She gave a half laugh, half sob. "Wouldn't that be glorious."

Phoebe jumped onto her mother's lap, kneaded her front paws a few times, and settled into a furry curl. Mum stroked the feline, breaking her own rule of no pets allowed at the table.

"Partly I stayed because my own cursed stubbornness wouldn't let me leave. In that way I'm like your grandfather. I wanted to prove to every disbeliever and doubter that I'd been violated and maligned, and I assumed I was suggesting the opposite if I fled. But I was foolish. There's no proof either way, and Kenton is convincing.

Even our family friends surely had doubts about what exactly occurred, but I *swear* I've always told the whole truth." She reached out and Anne took her hand. "And it doesn't matter. I should have put you ahead of my pride and taken you away. I would have, if I'd thought being here was so unbearable. And why wouldn't it be?" A tear trickled down her face, which she released Anne's hand to brush away.

Anne shook her head, suddenly contrite. "I might not be as strong and proud as I am if you'd taken me away. And sometimes, in my more charitable moods," she admitted, "I'm grateful for a fear that I've inherited some of Kenton's nefariousness. It makes me strive to be a good person." She paused. "Still, if I could have one wish, he deserves a comeuppance."

Her mother nodded.

Anne got up, went to her mother, and knelt beside her. She drew in a deep breath, steeled herself then said, "I'd like to know *exactly* how it happened, if you can tell me. You've never said, and I didn't want to force your remembering. But how were you even in that position?"

Her mother gazed down at Phoebe and smoothed the cat's sleek fur. Waited. Phoebe's purr melded with the hiss of the burning coal in the stove.

"There was no flirtation." Her mother stroked the cat with long, even glides of her hand. "I'd seen him eyeing me on the street, and in a shop or two, but I told myself I was being a ninny and imagining things. I was barely eighteen, and shy. He was married and had five children, one a newborn! I was picking blackberries, and he came upon me while riding. Dismounted and…asked for a taste." Mum palmed Anne's hand and grimaced. "Then he said he had a craving for more than berries."

Her blonde head bent, and a fat tear plopped atop Phoebe's head. The cat flicked its ears, shook, and jumped down. Anne wrapped her arms around her mother, who rested the side of her head against the top of Anne's, and the rest of the story was whispered, raw, told in a strained voice that made Anne's chest ache. It had been violent.

"I fought. When he forced me down, I grabbed a rock and struck him."

"I hope you hurt him."

Anne's mother raised her head and leaned back to look at her. Anne dropped her encircling arm, and her mum swiped her fingers under her eyes and over wet cheeks. "He laughed it off, said he'd known I had spirit under all my demure ways. But I left a scar. Here." She pointed to the crest of her left cheekbone.

"Even with that evidence you weren't believed?"

"By the time I accused him, it was healed and he had a tale to explain it. Kenton never said anything other than it wasn't rape. Most of the community decided I'd flirted and things got out of hand, that I'd brought it on myself and then been sorry. They actually admired Kenton for his restraint when I accused him. But he left Buttermere, and it was three years before he returned. Father threatened him, and I think Kenton believed him. He never bothered me again." Her mum's eyes narrowed as if trying to sharpen her vision of those distant years. "Or maybe he heard my father had given me a pistol to carry in my medical bag."

Anne had her own pistol, given to her by her mother when she'd begun making independent visits to patient homes; Mum had made her promise to carry it. But now she shuddered. She remembered her grandfather warning her, "Never trust an aristocrat, Annie." He'd say it whenever they encountered Kenton at Sunday service or on the road. That and, "That one's going to hell."

Anne got up and reseated herself in a chair. Her mother gave her a watery glance, and Anne knew she was regretting keeping them in Buttermere. But years of caring for people whose lives had gone topsy-turvy in an instant had taught Anne an important lesson: No one knows what the future holds. And it's all too easy to look back and regret one's decisions.

Her mother had done the right thing, she was suddenly sure. She had been raised by a doting parent and grandparents. She'd been safe, had chosen work she loved, and had learned so much from Edwin. She thought herself a person of high morals and good character, and her upbringing here had formed those qualities. Mum might have regrets for herself, but she needn't regret raising her daughter in Buttermere. Especially not when Anne recalled what Faye Elmore had said almost a month before, and how highly Edwin always spoke of her mother.

"If it helps, I think there are plenty who believe you were truthful, Mum, even if they don't speak up. I know Edwin does." The thought made Anne feel a little better, both about herself and what she'd endured and what her mother had decided. But the thought also made her ask another question she'd always wondered. "Mum, is the attack why you never married?"

"No." Her mother shook her head. "Maybe. Or maybe I've just never met the right man."

The right man. Anne's mind filled suddenly with the image of Peter Matthews. Was that foolish?

"Do you really think Carter believes Kenton raped me?"

Mum's question pulled Anne back from her musing. The crests of Mum's cheeks had gone bright red, and Anne gave an emphatic nod. "I know he does."

"He's unceasingly respectful, never the least bit disparaging," her mother admitted. "I've always liked him for that."

"He's a good man," Anne agreed. Her mother's glowing cheeks weren't fading, though. Could the thought of *Edwin* be making her blush? Why had Anne never considered Edwin for her? She felt foolish and blind.

"The two of you might make a good match," she suggested.

Her mother's eyes went wide. "Heavens, no! I'm older."

"Not by much," Anne scoffed. "I think he's thirty-four."

"You don't consider nine years much?"

"No one looks askance when the man is nine years older," Anne said. "Think of the Elmores. And why should it matter, Mum? Besides, you're very youthful."

"Most likely not youthful enough to give him children, and every man wants children."

"You don't know that," Anne said. Had her mother already considered this? "I have no idea whether he wants children, but given the big-hearted man he is, if he did and he couldn't have his own, I think Edwin Carter would happily adopt a parentless child. And it never occurred to me before, but he is awfully attentive whenever the two of you are together."

"He's asked me to dinner on a couple occasions," Mum confessed. "And several times to take an afternoon drive with him."

Anne was shocked. How could she have failed to see that the two were attracted to each other? Edwin had never even hinted! Excitement surged into her chest, and her lungs worked like she'd just run a race.

"I declined the invitations," her mother said, but her eyes held the same look as Phoebe's when she begged for a special tidbit. She pressed her palms to her cheeks. "I feel self-conscious around him. Like a schoolgirl."

"Mum, it doesn't matter that you're older than Edwin. Isn't how *he* feels the important thing? You owe it to yourself to give him a chance. Get to know each other in a more personal way."

Her mother's gaze dropped to her lap, but a slow smile curved her lips. After a moment, the expression faded and she gave Anne a no-nonsense look. "I sense you want to help, but you've helped enough. I'll look after that part of my life myself."

Anne blinked and couldn't resist a small tease. "I certainly hope you do."

She collected their dishes and set them in the sink; then she heard her mother's rustling skirt and an arm came around her back. Her mother hugged her, the sides of their heads touching, and said, "You took me by surprise before, but Mr. Matthews...he's the first person I've ever heard of recovering from pyemia. It makes me think he's here for a special reason."

Anne wanted to believe that was true.

CHAPTER EIGHTEEN

Anne studied the bolts of cloth shelved in the back corner of Danvers Retail. She'd narrowed her choices down to a dark green, sapphire, and ruby plaid; a serviceable brown with narrow, gold-colored stripes; or a Royal Navy blue on white baroque pattern. The brown and gold would probably look best with her hair, but she preferred the jewel-like colors of the plaid. Since Peter's dramatic improvement two days ago, she'd been bursting with happiness. Somehow, buying fabric and making a beauteous new frock seemed the perfect way to celebrate. She wanted to dazzle Peter with it, too.

A child's excited voice made Anne glance up to see Belinda and her children entering the store, Richard Thorpe close behind. The latter was the breeder and trainer of Viscount Kenton's steeplechasers, and the son of his stable master. Anne tucked herself behind a segment of shelving to stay hidden. After their last meeting, she didn't know how her next exchange with her complicated and contrary half-sister would go, and she didn't want to find out now. She'd been enjoying herself.

Thorpe had grown up on Kenton's estates, Anne remembered. He and Belinda would have known each other all their lives. Thorpe might well have been a childhood playmate of Belinda, her brothers and sisters. He likely had been their constant riding companion.

"Take your time, Henry," Thorpe said, waving toward the sweets display. "A man should never hurry important decisions."

The boy flew to the row of jars arranged along the counter next to a scale: humbugs, barley sugars, fruit pastilles, toffee, and other sweets. Thorpe, and Belinda holding Rebecca, followed him to the counter.

"Good day, Mrs. Jennett, Mr. Thorpe," said Mr. Danvers, giving them a stern nod.

"Good day," Thorpe returned. "Give young Henry an ounce of whatever he wants, and I'll take an ounce of the humbugs."

Mr. Danvers weighed out an ounce of the peppermint-flavored sweets, wrapped them in paper, and handed them over. "Well then, young Henry," he said, turning to the boy. He leaned over the counter and gave a big smile. "What tickles your fancy, lad?"

The alteration in the shopkeeper's tone and demeanor was marked, going from strict headmaster to benevolent grandfather, a change so pronounced it turned Anne from curious to engrossed. With much excitement on Henry's part, the boy and Danvers began discussing available flavors of fruit pastilles.

Thorpe turned to Belinda. With his broad back effectively blocking the shopkeeper's view, the two fixed their regard on each other, and Thorpe opened a corner of his package and tilted it toward her. "I hope you'll allow me to treat you as well?"

Anne's half-sister widened her eyes and smacked her lips, and right before Anne's eyes Belinda became a woman quite unlike the one Anne had always seen before. Tipping forward, Belinda glanced into the package and, without altering her tilted posture, met Thorpe's gaze. "I'd be delighted—if you'd be so kind, sir?"

Thorpe seemed to take forever removing his glove. Finally barehanded, he retrieved a sweet and offered it. Belinda took it from his palm with lingering fingers, lifted the candy and slowly placed it in her mouth.

Shock hit Anne like she'd dropped through thin ice into freezing water. There was no mistaking the flirtatious intent here. Poor Mr. Jennett! He was so devoted to his wife and children. Countless times Anne had watched him seek Belinda's gaze from the pulpit, send her a loving smile, and then give his son a wink. And she had given up an entire way of life to be his wife, so she must have been in love. Yet, Anne couldn't interpret what she saw here as anything other than inappropriate.

Thorpe bent a little closer and said something in a low voice—too low for Anne to hear. Belinda laughed, and her face and voice both reflected true happiness. Amazement wiped away every other emotion in Anne. Belinda had always struck her as unusually restrained, yet now her face was open and shining, and her eyes sparkled. She looked…lovely.

The shop door opened. Faces composed, Thorpe and Belinda turned back to the counter, where Mr. Danvers was handing Henry his selected package of sweets. "Good day, Mrs. Elmore," the shopkeeper called.

"Good day to you," replied the woman entering the store. "I've come to have a look at your ribbon."

Faye Elmore's gaze passed over Thorpe and Belinda, who regarded her in return. Belinda smiled, but Mrs. Elmore just gave a short nod. Belinda's expression stiffened, and Anne bit back surprise. She had seen many use that same civil but hardly welcoming greeting to her half-sister, but she'd never drawn the correct conclusion. Somehow, after her exchange with Belinda at the rectory and today's observation of a different, carefree woman, Anne now understood. That usual expression of cool disdain, that austere manner, weren't her half-sister's natural way. Could it be that, rather than cold and arrogant, Belinda was protecting herself? Was she girding her warmer, more vulnerable self against ostracism, much as Anne protected herself from those who believed Kenton's version of her conception? In this, it seemed, she and Belinda were similar.

Faye Elmore rounded the aisle and spotted Anne. "Miss Albright!" she sang out. "How nice to see you. I wanted to thank you for sending the new thorn-apple home with Michael. I feel nervous when there's none in the house."

"You're welcome," Anne said quickly. "We received a shipment, so we've plenty again."

A glance at Belinda showed an alarmed look, then anger and resentment. Then Anne's half-sister whirled away, and Anne knew it'd be best to finish her shopping and leave the store.

CHAPTER NINETEEN

Peter lay on his back, a smooth, semi-heavy river rock clasped in his hand. Straight-armed, he lifted the rock overhead then slowly lowered it. Carter had given him the rock and suggested he engage in what exercise he could tolerate. The surgeon had supplied Peter with a pair of loose-fitting pants and shirt and told him to stop thinking of himself as an invalid, which a frustrated Peter had become prone to doing after the pyemia; he was at a point where he could and should concentrate on recuperating.

It was over a month since he'd been shot, a week since he'd rallied from the grip of pyemia. His wound was healing. His bone was knitting. He still had the occasional fever, but the intensity was mild compared to the suppurative fever, and the pain in his back had improved enough he could usually ignore it. His head was better, too, the spinning sensation resolved, the throbbing no longer severe. Now, instead of pain and dizziness and headache, it was simple weakness that plagued him. The pyemia had stripped away his strength and stamina.

Peter skimmed his hand down his trunk and felt the bumpy protrusion of ribs. His unaccustomed leanness and weakness made him feel he inhabited a stranger's body. Anne assured him he'd soon be back to his former mountaineering strength, though. She and Mrs. Pettigrew plied him with food, harangued him to eat. He did his best.

He turned his head at the sound of footsteps.

"Good day, sir," Owen Weaver said from the doorway of the convalescent room—a different Owen Weaver than he'd sent off to do his investigating, now with neatly trimmed hair and beard. Even with the empty, pinned-up sleeve of his missing arm, the young war veteran looked like a man Peter would want at his side in a fight.

"You're back! Come in, come in." Peter waved young Weaver into the room, sat up, and stuffed a pillow between his back and the iron headboard.

"I'm happy to see you're recovering," Weaver said, advancing.

"Indeed I am. Now tell me...have you caught my attacker?" It had almost been too much to hope for when he'd hired the constable's son, but young Weaver's last post had said he'd identified a plausible suspect, and certainly no attacks had occurred while Peter lay vulnerable in Buttermere.

Weaver took the cushioned chair but didn't sink back into it. He sat on the edge, bent forward, legs spread, hat held between his knees. "I wish I could tell you that, sir, but I can't. He disappeared. After searching high and low the whole of North Yorkshire, I thought it wise to look for him here. It's always possible he had second thoughts about your identity and decided to find out for certain who he'd shot."

Peter's heart gave a hard thump. "Bloody hell." Was someone lying in wait now, ready for the day he left this surgery and was once again exposed and alone? He'd been focused too much on his physical condition, Arthur's troubles, and his unexpected feelings for Anne, and stopped worrying about how he'd arrived in this position. That had to change.

"I've no evidence he's here," young Weaver continued, "but I've good reason to think he's the culprit, and he's in the wind."

"He's one of the miners?"

Weaver gave a nod. "A man named John Monroe."

Peter searched his memory. The name meant nothing to him.

"When I arrived in Cliff Gate, there were bad feelings and stirred tempers aplenty. Monroe's the ringleader of the angriest lot, who speak out against you. By far the most damning thing is that Monroe was gone from Cliff Gate—supposedly looking for work—every time you were attacked. He was away when I arrived, in fact. The day he returned he heard I was nosing about and disappeared again before I could question him. I considered others, your partner Hardesty included, but Monroe was the only one out of town at the crucial times." Weaver shrugged a shoulder. "I suppose your partner isn't fully cleared, since you think he'd hire someone to do the dirty work."

"Is Hardesty still in Cliff Gate?"

"Gone back to London, sir. I think the fog of ill will in Cliff Gate became intolerable for him." Weaver paused. "I thought to search the Buttermere-Borrowdale-Keswick area for Monroe, but I could go to London if you think that better. Follow Hardesty and see if he meets up with anyone unusual. Perhaps even Monroe."

"My man of business made discreet inquiries, and he believes the mine closure made Hardesty's financial situation uncomfortable but not desperate," Peter said, "so my suspicion of him is even lower than it was. Plus, I had a letter from Lawton. He thinks he has a solution for the colliery. The miners will begin shoring up the unstable areas as soon as supplies arrive. He's starting work on a new ventilation shaft as well. There won't be any coal production until the mine is secure, but the men will be back to work and Hardesty's income will follow as soon as repairs are completed."

"Yes, I spoke with Lawton," Weaver remarked. "He said to tell you he's sure now that his ideas will work."

"Excellent. I don't like knowing the man responsible for my attacks may never be brought to justice, but I'd be pleased if they were to stop. There might be nothing else to be done."

"Don't say that," Weaver admonished. "I'm not done yet. And don't you relax, either. Monroe could be here and completely unaware of the situation at Bellow Hill."

"You're right," Peter admitted, as much as he wished it weren't so. He reached under his mattress and tugged out his money pouch. "I'm paying you what's owed so far, but we're not done. Keep looking for Monroe, just as you suggested."

Weaver gave an emphatic nod. "Yes, sir."

"Now, it's been…how many days?"

"Thirty-nine."

Peter nodded and counted out what was owed.

Weaver pocketed the coins and rubbed the backs of his fingers along his jaw. "Sir, I've been thinking. Once this job is completed, I've got to find steady employment of a kind a one-armed man can do." His forehead creased. "I seem well-suited to this type of work, and I've enjoyed it. Do you think there'd be need for such investigative service in London?"

Peter thought a moment. "I do. I'll write a letter of recommendation and a list of my friends and associates whom you should apprise of your services."

Weaver's forehead smoothed. "Thank you, sir. There's nothing for me here, and from what I gather London has a surplus of veterans looking for a position, most not finding one. I appreciate your help."

Peter nodded. Owen Weaver was smart and capable. When he'd hired the young veteran, neither of them had imagined the job might lead to a vocation. Perhaps something good had come from being shot after all.

"Let's hope you find Monroe. His capture would be a superb beginning for this venture."

The constable's son grinned. "I'll do my best. And I'll check in with you every few days. Any idea how much longer you'll be staying in Buttermere?"

"I'm mending but not quite ready for travel to North Yorkshire," Peter admitted. He fiddled with the stone in his hand. Kenton was expected back any day now. He'd want Peter to complete his recuperation at Pennyton Park, but how could he stay there, wondering whether his godfather was a rapist? And he had to reveal his lie to Anne, which meant Peter's prevarications were headed for an imminent reckoning.

"However I may be moving to other accommodations," Peter said.

Weaver nodded and settled his hat onto his head. "My father will be able to get word to me if there's need."

The two said farewell, and Peter was left with his thoughts as the constable's son exited. He didn't think Anne would mind the omission of his true identity as much as she'd hate the concealment of his connection to Kenton, so he needed to tell her, soon, before his godfather returned.

What if she didn't understand? Became angry or hurt? What if she didn't forgive him?

Cold stole into his chest. His heart felt brittle, like one hard beat would make it shatter.

~

For two days following young Weaver's visit, Peter applied himself to eating and careful exercise as if he were planning to summit one of the big peaks. During times of rest he puzzled over how to tell Anne who he was without destroying her liking, trust, and what he believed to be warmer feelings. He *had* to be right about that, didn't he? Because he felt the same.

When Anne brought a cane and said it was time he trekked outside, it seemed nearly as daunting an expedition as up a slope of Mont Blanc. Peter was eager, but he found the walk a challenge. He concentrated on the placement of his cane and his feet, and Anne stayed at his side, ready to add her support if needed. But that wasn't going to happen. His pride demanded it.

Through the surgery and out into the front garden he went. He paused once to catch his breath and gaze at the previously unseen sunny-side of his blue hydrangea bush, which was so full of midsummer blooms it looked like a giant bouquet. Then he proceeded on to the two chairs and small table Michael had grouped under a tree, and he even managed to ease himself down to the seat, rather than dropping onto it.

Beaming, Anne took the other chair. "You've improved."

"I'm still getting fevers," he complained. He was tired of being sick.

Anne shrugged. "They're mild and growing less frequent. You're recovering."

Peter heard the back door of the house slam, and Michael Elmore came around the corner carrying two glasses. The youth walked across the yard and set the drinks on the table. "Mrs. Pettigrew thought you'd like some lemonade."

"Thank you. It's exactly what I need." Peter picked up his glass and drained half of it. Then he told Anne, "He beat me at backgammon yesterday." He gestured toward Michael with his glass. A grin split the youth's face as he shoved his hands into his pockets.

"You must be a good player," Anne said.

Michael flushed and, with a lingering look at Anne, headed back to the surgery.

Peter extended his legs and watched Anne stretch the long column of her throat to drink. He suspected that both he and the boy admired Anne in the same way, albeit Michael with the simplicity of youth. The boy was probably head-over-heels. Not that Peter himself wasn't fairly close.

Anne regarded him over her glass. "It really is remarkable the progress you've made."

"Really?" Peter said.

"Yes, that you even survived the pyemia… I've never seen it, and Mr. Carter says it's extremely rare. He said he read an account that suggests only two in a hundred recover."

A shiver ran down Peter's spine. Why him? Why had he been so lucky?

Looking at Anne, he thought he knew.

She must have read the look in his eye, for she blushed. "I'm happy for you, and I'm glad I played a small part, but Mr. Carter and I have so little control. Certainly not over infections of that type. So few recover."

Peter saw the sadness in her face. "I know we talked about this, but it's a wonder to me. How *do* you go on? How do you stay optimistic when there's so much death?"

Anne considered her folded hands for a moment and then looked up, her eyes golden—a trick of the light or an inner radiance, Peter didn't know, but he had to catch his breath and couldn't look away. Every moment seemed to increase his attraction to her. She was so different from Louisa, from what he'd once believed he wanted, but...

"What other choice is there?"

Peter said nothing.

"Sometimes not much can be done, but in those cases I do my best to ease suffering. When a patient is dying, I keep the person physically comfortable and calm, encourage them and their loved ones to make amends and forgive each other. I reassure them and try to relieve their fear. And when the passing is peaceful, I'm content that I helped. I focus on that and not on the failures. At least, that's what I attempt to do."

Wise, Peter thought. And her work sounded fulfilling. He'd give almost anything for an opportunity to exchange a few last words with his parents, a moment in which to discuss their differences and put their failures to rest. Or to have additional time with Louisa. For a moment he relived that night, diving into the cold water again and again until something, perhaps his mother's or father's spirit, warned him not to try again. Numb with cold, a raw mass of desolation, exhaustion and pain, he'd collapsed. Cheek pressed to the muddy bank, he'd cursed the dark and raging water beside him.

Anne continued. "I think God is pleased when I make someone's passing a bit easier. Everyone needs someone to hold on to sometimes. And I like being that, giving that."

She fell silent as Peter nodded. He wondered if her experiences with her mother and Kenton had led her to this place of giving. Or was it her experiences with the people of Buttermere? One thing was clear, though: Anne was thoughtful and kind, and she lived the most admirable, worthwhile life.

Was his own life admirable? Peter wondered. According to his parents, living an exemplary life meant fulfilling obligations that stretched back generations before his birth and would continue for generations after he died. He'd tried to do that for years now, but after being shot on the road to Buttermere those ambitions seemed emptier than ever. He was increasingly pleased by the attempts he'd made to improve others' lives, like what he was doing at the mine. Not the money he would make from it, or the estates he could maintain, but the people he could affect. It was all about the people.

He glanced over at Anne, feeling singularly at ease with her. He could admit it now more than ever, this shared approval and warm liking...and yes, a tremendous, lusty desire that went beyond any other he'd ever known. Even more than with Louisa. As perfect as she had been for the life he'd intended, he hadn't felt *this* with her.

It was so strange. If he'd broached with them the idea of marrying Anne, his parents would have been strongly opposed. They wouldn't have considered her refined enough to be a proper viscountess, wouldn't have seen her furthering the family and title and estates in any way. Except, the idea of their disapproval didn't flatten Peter anymore. He could best help future Jennetts by doing what was right, or by doing what made him happy. His parents had never learned what he had: there was far more to life than attaining money and position, collecting accolades, and even summiting mountain tops. A person had one life to live, and all were ultimately judged by the good they'd done, and by how much they'd loved the life they led.

A breeze came up, making the leafy canopy overhead rustle. Peter looked at Anne and murmured, "You—the way you live life—has made me question the way I've spent mine."

Her lips parted, and she looked distraught. Her hand reached out, hovering between them. "Oh, no, that can't be!"

He shook his head, trying to help her see he meant it as an admirable thing, wishing he could drop the pretense of his false identity. "No, it's all right. My...management has helped a few people become or stay financially secure, and I've stabilized Lord Easterbrook's estate, but that's not enough."

Anne stared at him. "I think you forget how important financial security is. Your employer, and the people who work for him, depend on you. I'm certain they appreciate all you've done. As must their families!"

"Yes," Peter acknowledged. "I've helped expand Lord Easterbrook's holdings and thereby provided many livings. That *is* important, and I wouldn't change it. But you give something beyond measure. I've watched and listened. The times you hold someone's hand at the worst moment of their life…well, when you do, you hold *them*. Their spirit. I can't imagine a more fulfilling act. And you did it with me."

Her gaze grew pensive and hopeful, as if she sensed their connection and wanted it confirmed as much as he did. But she said nothing. Why did she say nothing? Was he imagining this connection, then? Was he imagining the pull between them, and it had simply been her kind generosity of spirit, something she offered to everyone who needed her?

"For you," he suggested, "such moments are the reward?"

"Yes. It's a privilege and an honor," she agreed. "To receive the gift of trust? It's not something to be undervalued."

Peter shook his head. "No. I'd like to find that kind of fulfillment, too. Touching hearts, and in the process having mine touched as well."

Could she see what he was saying? He wanted to touch *her* heart. He wanted to live a life that would make him happy.

Anne offered her hand, and he took it. It felt slim, strong, and warm, and a tingle raced up his arm. But then she said something that knocked him backward again.

"The past few days you've been studying those books you sent away for. I think maybe, when you're immersed in architecture, your heart fills with the passion you're seeking." She placed her free hand on his chest, palm centered over his heart. The organ fluttered, and his thorax grew warm as if he'd just summited Mount Elbrus, opened his arms wide, and been filled with the wonder and joy of being alive. "Perhaps you should go back to it. You certainly have the skill—or could obtain it—to create places that uplift the heart."

A vision formed in Peter's head of people streaming into a magnificent museum or astonishing concert hall, or a safe place of work or a beloved home—something that combined his passions wholly and uniquely and that bettered people's lives. He couldn't imagine pursuing such happiness. But why couldn't he? People would eventually accept that a viscount had a hobby he indulged that brought about joy for other people, just as they'd eventually accept the fact that he had married a young woman born out of wedlock, a brilliant and focused young woman who—

A bolt of horror suddenly struck and knotted Peter's stomach. He was planning a future and he didn't even know where Anne stood with Snow. Or with Carter. For all his worrying about how she'd take his half-truths about his identity, and his thoughts of making her happy, he'd never got up the courage to reveal the truth or ask the disposition of her hand.

"An even deeper connection will be the one you have with your children," Anne continued. "I can see in your eyes what kind of father you will be. They will own your heart. And they will give you theirs."

Would they? Peter was suddenly unsure. His own upbringing—a fairly standard one, going by his conversations with peers—had separated him and his parents. Yet, would it have to be that way? He couldn't imagine Anne allowing her children to live apart from her as he himself had lived apart from his mother during his school years.

"What about you?" He couldn't go another day wondering and not knowing. "Are you going to marry Snow?"

Anne's eyes widened—those marvelous amber eyes— and her shoulders moved as she took a deep breath. "No. I told him last week. I..."

Relief surged through Peter, and then the deepest sort of satisfaction. But then Anne withdrew her hand from his chest as if she'd been stung, and the air in Peter's lungs seemed to follow. He coughed weakly. Anne's eyes followed, in the distance, a horse and rider racing across the open land northeast of the surgery.

"That looks like Mr. Thorpe," she said, seeming flustered. "He's in charge of breeding and training Kenton's hunters and steeplechasers. Summers he builds their stamina on our fells. One named Bright Penny took third at last year's Grand National."

Yes, Peter knew Thorpe. This was the man Arthur feared was tempting Belinda, though of course that was foolishness. He'd most recently renewed his acquaintance with the horseman at Aintree, where he'd watched the race with Kenton. Treewick Hall's own stable now counted a Pennyton hunter among its residents, and of the four hunters Peter owned, Halfpenny was the biggest jumper.

Would Thorpe turn in their direction? Peter couldn't greet him now, not with Anne here. The horseman would unknowingly betray Peter's secret: that he was Viscount Easterbrook.

"Look, he's going to jump," Anne said.

The gray rock wall she pointed to, higher than most, abutted the road. Thorpe, on a fine black that looked like it could run all day, pushed straight toward it. Head extended, tail streaming, and neat as a Grand National winner, the black sailed over. Thorpe pulled up and turned in the direction of the surgery at a trot.

"I'm ready to go in," Peter said.

"Are you sure?" Anne asked.

"I am."

Urgency gave Peter strength and made him steady, and he got to his feet without Anne's assistance. She raised her eyebrows but positioned herself beside him without further comment, and they headed back to the house. Peter used his cane and pushed himself as fast as he dared, but he was still slow. Slow, but fast enough. When he checked the road, he saw he'd be inside before Thorpe got close enough to recognize him.

The porch. Thank God. He needed to get better. He'd begun to exercise, but he needed to do more. How long before he sat his horse again?

"I hope," he said, "Snow's giving Red enough exercise."

Anne held the door and gave him a look of such innocence Peter knew she was about to make a joke. "You could ask Michael to bring him by for a visit. Perhaps we could all have tea. I'll set up a table in the horse shed."

She was teasing, but a sudden longing to see Red struck.

"That would be nice," he said. "Red particularly likes lemon cake." Then Peter entered the surgery, knowing that sooner rather than later he'd have to tell Anne Albright who he really was, and he needed to do that before he told her how he felt. He'd only barely dodged the bullet of Richard Thorpe.

CHAPTER TWENTY

It was another busy day of scheduled patient examinations, and Anne accompanied Sarah Tennant and her son to the front door as they left the surgery. Elmer was the last of the morning patients. Edwin had examined the boy's arm and pronounced it healing well, and Anne had padded and re-splinted the fractured appendage after applying a lotion she hoped would alleviate his discomfort.

"Does it feel better?" she asked. "Less itchy?"

The twelve-year-old shrugged. He raised his splinted arm and glared at it. "Two more weeks!" His voice held all the disgruntled dismay of a boy who'd found an empty stocking on Christmas.

Anne pushed against the door just as it swung open. The unexpected loss of support made her stumble forward—right against the broad chest of Peter Matthews, who gripped her arms, his cane clattering against the floorboards.

"Miss Albright!"

For a moment Anne's surprise held her mute and immobile. Of the two of them, he should have been the wobbly one, yet *he* steadied *her*. Then he grinned.

He wasn't one for grinning, and it transformed him. He was always handsome, Anne knew, but the warmth and humor that filled his face these days—that sparkled in his eyes since he'd begun rehabilitative exercises—made everything else fade away. They stood so close. Close enough for her to see the dark gray rim that encircled the blue irises of his eyes and smell the peppermint on his breath.

Since their conversation outside five days ago, they had not talked about how much closer they felt, but she knew they both did. They'd shared parts of themselves they protected and secreted away from everyone else, and found not merely acceptance but mutual admiration. That closeness proved she'd been right to refuse Andrew. Her feelings for Peter were so much more than the warmth of friendship. Of course, he hadn't made any declarations of love or anything, but he was increasingly focused on his health, working hard, determined to improve. She liked to think that he would acknowledge their connection when he was fully recovered. His color had bettered and every day he seemed stronger, but he was far from returned to full health and vigor. He was just well enough to have become frustrated with his slow recovery.

Her hands splayed against his chest. Heat raced up her arms, making her heart gallop. Then Peter eased her away, not quite releasing her until she took a step back. A garbled laugh croaked from her throat, and she side-stepped toward the porch rail.

"Pardon me, Mr. Matthews," she said. Relief and disappointment at the increased distance between them cooled her overheated flesh.

"Sir?"

Elmer had snagged Peter's attention, offering his dropped cane. Peter accepted the walking aid and now, elbow locked, took advantage of its support. "Thank you. You must be the tree-climber from several weeks ago. How's the arm coming?"

The boy's eyebrows shot up and disappeared behind his tousled brown hair. "How did you know?"

Peter indicated the surgery with a tip of his head. "The day you fell, I was in the next room and heard all. The exact same thing happened to me when I was about your age."

"You fell out of a tree?" Elmer asked.

Peter gave a nod. "And broke my arm. How much longer until the splint comes off?"

Elmer scowled. "Two more weeks."

Peter drew a folded square of paper from his pocket. Anne had seen it before, when Peter offered her one of the peppermint candies he'd had Michael purchase yesterday on a trip to Danvers Retail. "Perhaps this will help."

He unfolded the paper and extended it. The boy reached out, then paused and looked at his mother.

"Thank the gentleman, son," Mrs. Tennant said.

Elmer barely had the words out before he had the candy in his mouth, lips pursed and sucking. Peter offered peppermints to Elmer's mother and Anne next, then rewrapped them and slipped them inside his coat. Mrs. Tennant expressed her own thanks, wished both Peter and Anne good-day, and ushered her son out and down the front path.

Peter held the door, waiting for Anne to enter the surgery in front of him. She passed through and stopped in the waiting area. Peter followed.

"How far did you walk?"

"To the stable-yard," he said. "I checked on Red and sat a spell visiting with Andrew Snow."

"Any dizziness or shortness of breath?"

"No. Mr. Snow seemed fit enough." Anne stared at him, then laughed, and then Peter answered her question in earnest. "No dizziness. A little shortness of breath, but it's getting better."

Dark circles shadowed the skin below Peter's eyes, and Anne allowed herself a moment's annoyance. She'd *told* him the stable-yard was too far to walk. Stubborn man!

"How is Red?" she asked.

"Enjoying the easy life. Snow is having a boy exercise him, but it's much less activity than he's accustomed to."

The sound of Edwin descending from the second floor had them both turning to the stairs. The surgeon called out, "Come on, let's eat," and strode toward the dining room where Mrs. Pettigrew would serve them luncheon. Peter had been using the dining room for meals the past several days, then after eating would retire to his room to nap. Today would be a good test, Anne decided. If the walk had been too exhausting, he wouldn't eat much.

He ate only half the portion of soup Mrs. Pettigrew served him, and a few bites of bread—less than half the amount Edwin, a man with a vigorous appetite, consumed in the same amount of time. Still, Peter made a humming noise when he tasted the first spoonful, his brows raised and his body tucked closer to his bowl. Anne counted that as a fairly good sign.

Edwin released his spoon into his empty bowl and pushed away from the table, chair scraping against the floor. "I'm off to attend Lady Kenton. It's time her sutures came out."

Anne nodded. She'd told him about the laudanum. He'd questioned the viscountess upon a follow-up visit, but Lady Kenton denied excessive use. Anne was not surprised by that. Carter had assured her he intended to pursue the matter in a different way.

"The supplies you ordered came in today's post," Anne told him. "I'll put everything away."

"The chloroform arrived intact?"

"Yes."

"Good. I may have to amputate Thomas Russell's toes." When Anne grimaced, Edwin added, "I think young Tom has taken over the majority of the farm work, so at least the family's survival is assured if the father can't work."

"What happened to his toes?" Peter asked.

"Russell has a circulatory impairment that's caused a dry gangrene. He's afflicted with diabetes. I've seen other patients with the condition who lost circulation to their feet. I'm of the opinion the two conditions are related."

Peter nodded, seeming to take this in. After Edwin left, Anne sat with him in companionable silence while they finished their tea.

At last he drained his cup, set it on its saucer and pushed the china away. "I'm going to the scullery and chat with Mrs. Pettigrew for a bit.

Perhaps convince her to sing a ditty or two. She's as entertaining as a music hall performer."

Anne laughed and stood. "All right. I'd best start putting the supplies away."

She went to the treatment room. After putting the room to rights after the morning's patients, she turned to restocking their tinctures, herbs, and medicinal agents. Sometime later, Peter joined her and settled onto the chair they kept for patients' relatives.

"Feeling better now that luncheon has settled and you've rested a bit?" Anne asked.

"I feel fine, and you needn't waste your breath with another lecture about overdoing it. Your frowns send a very clear message, and I already got one when I returned from my walk."

Anne pinched her lips in order to withhold a smile. "I see."

Peter stood, ambled over and watched her return a jar to its place. "I'm improving, enough so that I'm starting to feel restless." He shrugged. "I'm tired of reading and sketching, and my backgammon games with Michael don't happen often enough. I hope I'm not being a nuisance."

"Not at all." She pulled the next jar down and opened it.

"That smells like cinnamon."

Anne finished counting and looked up. "Cinnamon bark from Ceylon. It's best when it's very fresh, so we don't order large quantities."

"How about the leaves Tim Elmore smoked? Where did they come from?"

"Thorn-apple is found all over England." Anne waved a hand at the many jars and canisters shelved within the tall apothecary cupboard. The array of containers had a variety of tops: glass stoppers, corks, and wax seals. "We've medicinals from the Americas, India, all sorts of exotic places, but the majority are readily available in England or Europe. Some I collect myself."

"Really? You dry them? Make your own elixirs and tinctures?"

"Sometimes." She pointed to several side-by-side jars. "Those contain different forms of angelica: the root, dried leaves, and stewed and preserved stems and leaves. I collect it every summer and usually have enough to last the year. It's useful for a number of maladies."

Peter looked impressed. He asked a few more questions as she worked, and the time passed companionably. Just as she was finishing, the bell affixed to the front door jangled.

"Hello? Anyone here?"

A man's voice.

Anne hurried to the front and found a stranger perusing the room. In tall boots and a serviceable coat, with a horse she saw tied out front bearing full saddlebags, she guessed him to be a traveler.

"May I help you, sir?"

"Good day, ma'am. I hope so. I've run out of my tonic." He plunked an empty bottle of Dr. Perry's Emulsion on the table. "I'm worried by dyspepsia on occasion," he explained.

"Mr. Carter doesn't sell patent medicines," Anne said. "But Danvers Retail, just down the road, does."

The man seemed more interested in his surroundings than what she was saying. He strolled to the sick room door and gazed in.

"Sir?"

The man finally looked at her, but his gaze kept moving. Past her.

Ah. He was looking at Peter, who entered and stood beside her.

"Are you the doctor?" the stranger asked. His gaze raked Peter from head to toes.

"No."

The abruptness of Peter's answer surprised Anne. So did his expression—or lack of expression.

"Hmmph." The stranger swept his gaze back around the room, then picked up his empty bottle and waved it. "Your doctor should sell this. Save folks from wasting their time." Then he spun and left, the doorbell jangling in his wake.

Anne shrugged. "Well. He was a strange one."

Peter didn't comment. He gazed out the window, attention focused on the stranger. When he moved back, she realized how stiffly he'd been standing.

"Is everything all right?"

"I hope so. You forget I was shot, and he's the first stranger I've seen since I arrived here."

~

Peter watched the stranger mount and ride in the direction of Danvers Retail, a crawly sensation snaking down his neck and spine. The dyspeptic man's curiosity struck him as odd, and odd didn't sit well with him anymore. Oh, why hadn't he asked Owen Weaver for a description of Monroe when last they spoke? Weaver hadn't had any luck in the area, but that didn't mean his quarry wasn't eluding him.

Peter rubbed the back of his neck and filled his lungs with air. He hadn't considered his assailant might be bold enough to approach him mid-day, in the surgery. That was extremely unlikely, wasn't it? The stranger was probably no one to worry about. Still...should he relocate to his godfather's estate? Kenton was expected home in the next three or four days. Peter would unquestionably be safer at Pennyton, but he'd been enjoying ignoring the investigations that awaited him there.

His eyes went to Anne, who watched him with a tipped head.

"You should rest," she said, seeming to mistake his unease for fatigue. That relieved him of having to lie, since his recent activity *had* tired him, and when he said nothing she shrugged. He followed her back into the treatment room, where she retrieved what he called her bandage basket from the bottom of the large supply cupboard; in all those days of her sitting at his bedside, many times he'd been lulled to sleep with the quiet sounds and repetitive movement of her hands tearing and rolling strips of cloth.

"Keep me company for a while?" he asked. He couldn't help himself. No matter how much time she spent with him, it never seemed enough. "I'm weary but not sleepy."

She nodded and followed him back to his room, placed her basket on the ottoman and settled in the big upholstered chair.

Peter situated himself with the headboard and pillows against his back and swung his legs onto the bed. "I should have gone to Danvers Retail from the stable-yard. I'd like to give Mrs. Pettigrew a small gift. She's been very kind, asking what dishes I prefer, and trying to provide foods for which I've a fondness. Perhaps I'll walk down before supper."

Anne gave him a look, and he understood her message: *Stop being stupid.* Danvers Retail was at the far end of town. He'd just gotten back from walking to the stable-yard, and she'd advised him against that as well. And Lord knew he was tired from overexerting himself. Still, how else was he to check on the stranger who'd just come calling? Would he just have to wait for Owen Weaver to come back?

Tearing a strip from the fabric in her lap she said, "You could send Michael if you've an idea what to purchase. He got you those peppermints, and he'd be happy to do you another favor. He rushes through his chores so he'll have time to play backgammon with you before going home these days."

"He's a bright boy," Peter said. But that didn't make it appropriate for him to do Peter's snooping.

For a time, quiet reigned. Motes, likely cast-off from Anne's ripped fabric, floated in the afternoon sunshine that angled through the window. Peter exhaled, and every muscle went heavy and relaxed. Maybe he was being silly about the stranger. Maybe he should focus on other things, especially things he'd been putting off for far too long.

"I…had a thought," he said.

"Oh?" Anne glanced up.

"Yes." The rolling action of her slender fingers was mesmerizing. Peter was more tired than he'd thought, and looking into those eyes he just couldn't bring himself to tell her the truth. Not now. So he mentioned a different idea that had been in his head recently, an idea that might change a life like Anne did—for the better.

"We might sit down together each afternoon—you, me, and Michael—and read aloud from a novel. I borrowed *David Copperfield* from Carter, which I'm sure will engage the boy. I thought we might start with that."

Anne paused and glanced up. "You want to instill a love of reading in him."

Ha! How quickly she'd surmised that. Perhaps it was unsurprising, given their recent conversations. Seeing Michael every day had made him consider how best to help the youth, and he'd noticed a keen intellectual curiosity as well as a facility with board games. How better to feed that than with books?

"I could well imagine him following in Carter's footsteps with a little encouragement," he said.

Anne looked thoughtful. "You may inspire a love of learning in Michael, but his family could never afford to send him away for advanced schooling."

"Perhaps," Peter suggested slowly, "if Michael acquires the desire, an avenue will open." He intended to be the lad's benefactor, of course. The satisfaction he'd receive from vouching for the boy and financing his schooling would be great.

"I suppose the Elmores could appeal to Kenton," Anne mused, her hands frozen in her lap. "The viscount might sponsor Michael. But I can't bear to think of the boy and his family feeling beholden to that man."

"I'll recommend Michael to Lord Easterbrook," Peter said. "He's provided scholarships for some of his tenants' children in the past. I'm confident he'd help Michael, should the boy prove interested."

"Truly?" Anne resumed winding her bandage roll, the corners of her mouth turned up. "I forget sometimes that you work for a viscount of your own. He must be very kind if he has not complained about you being laid up here so long."

Peter thought fast. "The letter I received from the viscount's man of business included a note from Easterbrook. He's always been involved in the management of his estates, and he's enjoying his temporarily expanded role. He has the time right now, since Parliament will very soon be in recess."

"How exciting it would be if your viscount sponsored Michael," Anne said. "If he could avail himself of an advanced education, he could certainly apprentice with Mr. Carter. I too can imagine him being a surgeon or apothecary one day. Edwin is an excellent teacher. He's taught me everything I know—apart from what my mother taught me."

"And that is no mean amount of knowledge."

She glanced at him, smiled, then turned her eyes back to the work in her lap. "He's one of the best men I know. Part of the reason I've stayed in Buttermere is because of him. I wouldn't have the same opportunity anywhere else."

Peter felt a moment of unease. He'd convinced himself his fears of Carter as a suitor were foolish after the warm conversations he and Anne had lately shared, and after she hadn't mentioned him when she mentioned turning down Andrew Snow. But they had been interrupted by the appearance of Robert Thorpe. Was there something she just hadn't told him yet? Just as he had forgone telling her all?

"You've definitely accomplished a great deal together," he said. "I didn't know you, yet you made me feel safe from the start."

It was true. He didn't discount what Carter had done for him, but Anne was a critical force as well. *She* was the one who had been at his side every moment of his recovery. *She* was the one who made Carter's surgery as warm a place as it was. She was clearly special, both her mind and her passion for helping people, and he wondered at her fear of not being able to find a place anywhere else.

Anne smiled, but she didn't look up. "I'm glad."

"I..." He was thinking about the future again. If he moved to Kenton's estate, everything would change between the two of them. But perhaps he could learn how to better proceed, ask questions that would allow him to say the right things to smooth over his mistakes. "I hope you'll forgive my asking, but I've been thinking about your past and wondering about Viscount Kenton," he said. "You say he might help Michael, and that he has helped other people in the village. Has he supported you financially?" His face burned suddenly as he feared Anne's embarrassment. "Given your...connection, I mean."

Anne gave a fast, hard shake of her head and glanced up, lips a thin tight line. "He offered, but Mum refused."

"Ah," Peter said. "I can understand your mother not wanting any connection to him. I suppose you must feel the same. Even if you might gain from—"

Anne's head shot up. "A rapist and a liar? I worry far more about what he's given me already, what blood is running through my veins, than about what advantages I might be missing out on by avoiding the blackguard. I want nothing to do with him."

Peter saw how her hands squeezed the fabric roll, and he bit back astonishment. "You truly worry you might have inherited some despicable trait from him?"

"Of course." She looked up and stared into his eyes, but she didn't say anything else.

"I'm sorry," he said. "That you went through that."

"Probably for the best," Anne said, shrugging. Her eyes shuttered a bit. "Now I try to be always kind and honest—the opposite of him in all things." Her brows bunched, and her lips firmed. "I can't abide liars. A man who can't be honest with the world can't be honest with himself, and a man like that isn't worth knowing."

Her vehement words, as much as he agreed with them, delivered a cricket bat–blow to Peter's chest, and a soft groan slipped out of him. He rubbed his hand over the ache and wondered how he could tell her now that he'd been lying all this time. Now that he knew Anne and Carter, he was extremely sorry he'd withheld his identity in the first place. They never would have revealed his secret, on purpose or by accident.

And his relation to Kenton…

The ache grew.

Her voice roused him from his reflections. "Sometimes I regret not knowing my half-brothers and sisters, especially recently. Belinda and Mr. Jennett married four years ago. I see her frequently, even work with her on occasion, and…well, I… Ever since she helped with little Nan Blythe's birth, I've thought we might drop our barriers and perhaps develop a friendship. I think things are different for her than I realized."

Peter nodded, pleased. Such a relationship might even pull Belinda out of her malaise. Too, perhaps some mended fences could soften the blow of his two untruths. "I think you *should* be friends with Mrs. Jennett. You should at least be on speaking terms with all of the family."

Anne shook her head. "Not Kenton."

Peter couldn't help himself. "Have you ever even talked to him?" He just couldn't imagine his friend being the monster that Anne and her mother believed, and the idea that he would be anything but kind and thoughtful to a daughter seemed outlandish.

Anne looked a bit sheepish as she shook her head again. It surprised Peter, given the intensity of her rage only a few minutes before. "He's only in Buttermere a few months out of the year, and he's never actually admitted he fathered me. I've avoided him."

Peter sat up, feeling that perhaps here was a possibility. If maybe there was a mistake, if maybe there was a misunderstanding and he could get Anne and her father to make peace, perhaps she would forgive Peter for deceiving her. Perhaps there was still some explanation that made both Anne's mother and James Kenton good people.

Anne hesitated and looked uncertain, as if she were deciding something. She took a deep breath. "When I was a child, and even later, when I was old enough to understand and know better, I wanted him to love me. I never told anyone. I knew, if my mother or grandparents ever realized how I felt, they'd be very hurt. I knew it was something I *shouldn't* want. I knew it was wrong. But every time I saw him, I hoped. And every time he turned his eyes away, I filled with disappointment. Finally I matured enough and gained enough understanding that I didn't want his fatherly affection. Quite the opposite. I am appalled that I come from him. At the same time, I'm outraged that he's never acknowledged his paternity, as if he considers me below his notice or not up to the standard of his offspring."

She paused, her breathing fast and her color high. Peter waited. He could tell there was more.

Her expression became pained as she continued. "Except, when I think of confronting him, I have this great fear that, if he should confess to loving me, or wanting to love me, I'd be glad."

She released a great sigh, and his heart clenched. Dear Anne, to carry such a burden. He took her hands and drew them toward him. They were soft yet strong. So capable, so giving. They'd wiped away his sweat, bathed him, turned him, carried spoons to his mouth.

He rubbed his thumbs across her knuckles. "Like any other child, you wanted to be loved by your father. You have no reason to be ashamed by that. You're an adult now. Meeting with him won't happen the simple way you imagined it growing up. The situation between you is complicated. If he did declare paternal feelings for you, it would be your decision how to respond."

Her gaze searched his eyes and she gave a nod. After a moment he went on. "Trust me. You won't be surprised or appalled by your reactions to him. And you deserve the chance to express your feelings. At the very least you must declare your anger, expunge it instead of holding it inside. You deserve to have answers to your questions!"

She said nothing. Her gaze dropped to the floor, and Peter suddenly reconsidered his words. Was he selfishly forcing on her something she didn't want because it would perhaps solve his own worries? He didn't think so. She needed to vent her feelings to the man. He was her father! And if it helped provide a solution to Peter's problem, all the better. Maybe there was even a future that neither of them yet saw. Anne's heart was bigger than anyone's. Maybe she'd find a solution to her parentage that nobody could guess, would figure out why and forgive Peter for not revealing his true name and title, for hiding his association with Kenton. Was that too much to hope? He had to tell her soon, but perhaps first she might interact positively with her father. The falsehood would unquestionably hurt her, but perhaps there was relief to be found as well. Perhaps joy.

She was so lovely. With one finger, Peter lifted her chin. Hand sliding against the silk of her hair, he cupped the base of her head. Tested for resistance. Gave in to his wildest temptations.

With only the smallest pull she leaned toward him. He moved slowly, giving her the opportunity to balk, but she didn't. The scent of newly opened roses filled his head, and their lips met in a kiss unlike any he'd experienced. A kiss that made him forget all good intentions of staying in control and ignited a fire that swept through his belly, his chest, his limbs. All he wanted was to lay her on the bed and let their passions carry them away.

A little moan came from her throat and a shiver streaked down his spine. He slid a hand around her waist and drew her closer still. Her lips parted. Heart pounding, blood pulsing, he finally tasted her.

Yes.

He tasted and explored and kissed, and he found his eagerness matched by hers. A ferocious need filled him and cemented the bond he felt. Her hands slid down his back, up his chest. His skin tingled. His heart ballooned until it pressed against the cage of his ribs. He slid his mouth across her face and tasted the sweetness of her neck.

"Peter."

His name floated on a sigh, one word full of amazement and longing and pleasure, and Peter's body turned to rock—and not in a good way. He'd been reminded of his lie. She didn't know he was Peter Jennett, Viscount Easterbrook. He was taking advantage of her ignorance and making everything so much worse.

He drew back. God, his hands were shaking.

He dragged a hand down his face and exhaled with a gust. "I…I'm sorry. I…lost my reason for a minute. It won't happen again. Not until I'm no longer in your care and no longer in this house. With Carter coming back any time and Mrs. Pettigrew in the kitchen…"

She stared up at him, silent. God, she was beautiful. Her amber eyes gleamed, her mouth swollen from his kisses, her cheeks pink as the peonies outside the surgery's front door. Contrasting with her burnished hair, her skin looked like cream. He wanted to lick the scatter of tiny nutmeg-like freckles that bridged her nose.

Anne's chest rose with a large breath, her lips parting as she studied him. Then her breath rushed out. "Yes. I…This was wrong. Thank you. For stopping."

Her face flushed, she popped to her feet. He leaned back but made no move to rise, just lifted her basket, which she took before sweeping from the room. He hoped that she understood this was really for the best. He'd been wanting to kiss her for a very long time, but it couldn't happen again. Not until he told her everything.

He loved her. God, it was true. So this was the very least he could do for her. He and Anne would know a prodigious passion and defy all those narrow-minded peers who might challenge the perfect marriage of a viscount and woman bent on bringing comfort to the world. But it had to be done the right way at the right time.

CHAPTER TWENTY-ONE

All of a dither, Anne made her way to the kitchen and found it unoccupied. Mrs. Pettigrew's apron hung beside the door, which meant she'd gone out, thank goodness. Relieved to have the room to herself, Anne prepared tea and dropped into a chair at the table.

After the first sip of steaming brew, her shoulders loosened. She sighed and leaned against the hardwood chair back. Peter had *kissed* her. He hadn't planned it, she didn't think, but she was so glad he had. Her attraction and tenderness weren't one-sided. He felt the same things she did.

She cradled her steaming teacup, remembering and marveling. No one, not even Andrew Snow, with his professed devotion, had gazed at her the way Peter did, with a mix of happiness and longing, and no one else had ever made her feel so unique and special. She didn't know how she looked at him, if her face gentled the way his did, but she knew he was everything she'd ever imagined loving and more. She had never experienced desire until they kissed, either. Now she was tumbling straight into an overwhelming yearning.

How lucky she was. She'd feared that turning down Andrew might leave her alone forever. Instead, the man she met not only turned her blood to honey, he didn't look down on her for the circumstances of her parentage. She trusted him to the same degree she trusted Mum and Edwin, and—

He'd suggested she talk to Kenton. He was the first person to ever do that. Was that wise or foolish? And, was she brave enough? She'd always had questions for her father, but she'd never been able to confront him.

Peter said the plan was wise. That made her gather courage and bolster her resolve.

The kitchen door suddenly opened, surprising her. Edwin walked in, hung his cap on an empty peg, and rubbed his hands together. "Good. There's tea." He lifted the cloth covering whatever Mrs. Pettigrew had left in the middle of the table for them and said, "Mmm. My favorite." Scones made with dried apricots, Anne saw.

Edwin strode to the sink, worked the pump and washed his hands, then returned to the table with a plate and teacup. Anne slid the bowls of clotted cream and apricot jam closer. Edwin's obvious enjoyment as he availed himself of the snack amused her; the man never turned down an opportunity for food, yet stayed lean as a hungry cat. She couldn't help wondering if he and her mother would someday get together. It was all the more poignant a thought when she was still buzzing with love for Peter.

"God bless Mrs. Pettigrew," Edwin said, and Anne chuckled. "Anything unexpected occur while I was gone?"

"No," Anne said—too quickly. At Edwin's look she added, "How did Lady Kenton's wound look?"

"Healed. I removed the ligatures. She seemed distracted and… vague. I asked if she'd taken laudanum, and if she remembered how I'd asked her if she was taking it too often. She became agitated and said she'd only dosed herself in case the suture removal caused pain. I can't imagine her thinking I'd accept that. I tried to explain the deleterious effects of taking too much, as if they aren't obvious. She said she took only as much as required and I needn't concern myself." Edwin pulled off his spectacles, rubbed the red marks on either side of the bridge of his nose, and reseated the eyewear. "I said I wanted to help but I needed to understand the whole situation. I told her she could trust me. She gave me a look..." His shoulders and hands lifted, the way they did whenever he felt helpless.

"A look?" Anne encouraged.

"The only way I can describe it is contempt. We were in the sitting room along with her lady's maid. Lady Kenton stood, said, 'You needn't bother yourself,' and told her maid—Miss Brown, I think?—to see me to the door. Then Lady Kenton marched out."

"What will you do?" Anne asked. Edwin wasn't the type to let things be, not when he could help. Not until he had tried every tactic and done his best to perform his duty.

"She won't get any more laudanum from me, but that won't matter since it's on every apothecary's shelf." He shrugged. "I'll have to speak to Kenton once he's back."

Anne's stomach flipped. She would soon have the opportunity to speak to him as Peter suggested. Their conversation had made her want to look Kenton in the eye and ask all of her questions, but... could she muster the nerve?

Edwin's voice brought her back to the matter at hand—trying to help Lady Kenton. He was right to try, unkind as the viscountess might be to all of them.

"I have no idea how Kenton will react," Edwin admitted. "You don't know this, but I've done my best to keep my distance from the man. I'm hardly civil, and I've declined many dinner invitations. He finally stopped asking and let me know he doesn't care for my 'disagreeable disposition.' But when I think of him hurting—*raping*—your mother, I want to smash his arrogant face."

Anne felt warmth pour through her at Edwin's protective words regarding her mother. She'd always known Edwin sided with them, and now, having this conversation, she wished she hadn't promised Mum not to interfere. "I didn't realize. Does Mum know?"

Edwin frowned. "I doubt it. We've never discussed it."

Anne grasped the teapot handle and refilled their cups. She didn't speak until after she'd added milk and sugar to hers. "I'm sure Kenton knows why you've been rude, given your connection to our family. It means a lot that you've let him know how you feel. No one else has."

"I haven't done enough," Edwin muttered. "I don't know what Emma still retains from the horror of that experience, but I consider her the sweetest, kindest, and most honest woman I know."

"Yes." Her mum *was* the sweetest, kindest, and most honest woman in the world, and it was just wonderful that Edwin felt the same. "I'm lucky," Anne added as her heart squeezed. When she thought of her parentage, it was usually to deplore her father. She didn't appreciate often enough how fortunate she was to have such a wonderful mother.

They each took a couple more swallows of tea. Edwin broke the corner off another scone, spread it with cream and jam, and tossed it into his mouth.

"Mum and I had a talk about you recently," Anne said, throwing caution to the wind.

Edwin stopped chewing. He swallowed, hard, and sat up a little straighter. "About me?"

Anne nodded. "I know she's refused your invitations for walks and carriage rides, but if you offered another I think she might accept."

Above his neatly trimmed beard, Edwin's cheeks flushed cherry, and Anne had a sudden urge to laugh and clap her hands. Especially when his slow smile turned into an embarrassed grin. His eyes glinted.

"I'd given up," he admitted.

"Please," Anne begged, "don't do that."

"I won't," he agreed.

Still smiling, he placed the remainder of the broken scone on his plate and began to spread it with more cream and jam. He and Anne both fell silent, and Anne sipped her tea.

Please, Mum, be brave, she thought. More than anyone, her mother deserved love.

Edwin suddenly thumbed a smear of jam from the corner of his mouth and said something surprising. "Mr. Matthews is doing well. It won't be long before he'll be able to ride. It'd be best if he didn't leave until he's been free of fever for a full two weeks, but I don't know that he'll wait."

Anne's stomach flipped. Of course this was true. The day was fast approaching, and she wasn't ready. Their kiss had complicated everything. She needed time—*they* needed time—to see if this attraction would continue to grow. He'd stopped it for the sake of propriety, but now she regretted that. The kiss had been more than an exchange of desire. For her, at least, it had been a promise. An interrupted promise. A promise of the love she'd always hoped to find.

One with the perfect man.

CHAPTER TWENTY-TWO

There was something about walking the road between the surgery and home that drew Anne's mind to contemplation, and in the three days since Peter kissed her, little else filled her head. He was her first thought upon waking and her last thought at night. But they hadn't kissed again. Just talked with that usual warm camaraderie they shared. Talked and exchanged glances and unspoken feelings.

How right she'd been to refuse Andrew, who'd never generated a single daydream. When Peter kissed her, magic happened. The kind of magic that made a tight April rosebud burst into full, fragrant bloom. Magic that threw open her soul's doors and windows and gusted through like a warm summer breeze. Magic that teased and tempted and tortured.

The sound of approaching hoofbeats made her glance over her shoulder and pause. These long summer days the sun didn't set until nearly bedtime, and the late afternoon light was quite bright. She recognized the horse. Not only was it the most magnificent of all the Pennyton hunters she'd seen, but the stallion was Kenton's regular mount. She jerked her head around and doubled her pace toward home. He was back! And she wasn't ready to confront him.

His name assaulted her with each step. *Ken-ton. Ken-ton. Ken-ton.* She looked again. Yes, she knew that posture, ramrod straight, straighter and squarer than any mere mortal could manage, as if his skin were unyielding medieval armor. She pulled her shawl up to meet the edge of her bonnet, bent her head, and hoped he'd ride past.

Except...hadn't she decided to confront him? Peter had suggested she owed it to herself to speak her mind to him. Kenton had violated her mum without reprisal. He'd spread—or encouraged—lies about her innocent mother in order to protect himself. He was despicable, and Anne ached to tell him so. How would it feel to release the rage burning deep in her heart? To erase the lifelong lingering shame left by the childhood desire that he love her?

The sounds of his approach grew louder, and a sudden thought slowed her stride. Might she discover he concealed a special feeling for her, his illegitimate daughter? If that were the case, did that not make him vulnerable to her revenge? Did it not give her the means to hurt him in the name of avenging her mother? Her heart jumped into her throat. Part of her wanted him to know pain and misery, while another part despised such contemplation.

Shouldn't you at least try to talk to him? Will you forgive yourself if you don't?

There were certainly things she wanted to say.

Her feet slowed even more. The rhythms of her heart and lungs doubled, and each breath rasped in her ears, while the smack of her footsteps faded away along with the rustle of leaves and the chirp of the birds. Louder and louder came the clip-clop of hooves and huffs of equine breathing.

She stopped, fisted her hands, and turned. Twelve feet back, Kenton reined up his splendid gray stallion and sat easy, gazing down at her. A low-crowned hat shaded his eyes. His posture didn't change; it remained as rigid as ever.

Anne strode toward him, grabbed the gray's bridle, and spoke in a tone that warned patients' relatives they'd best pay attention or disaster would follow. "We need to talk."

Her heart thumped and her breath sawed in and out, but she held his gaze. Kenton's mouth went tight and he dismounted, fast; before she had a chance to prepare, he stood before her, a man of broad shoulders and hard eyes, a man emanating an aura of invincibility.

Anne released the bridle strap and stepped back. Kenton passed his reins over the gray's head and held them loosely. He didn't speak, and she didn't know how to start.

He sighed like he didn't have the time or desire to listen. "Well...?"

Anne's skin turned to ice, while her core blazed at his aristocratic impatience. She managed to say, "You're my father. I'd like to hear you acknowledge that."

"Would you really?"

His amber-eyed gaze inched over her face—eyes like Belinda's and Anne's own. She'd never been this close to him, watched his mouth form words, seen his white teeth. Icy needles cascaded over her shoulders and down her arms. Her mother had been this close and closer.

"What if I confirm your parentage, but in the telling you learn a few truths you don't want to know? Once a secret is revealed, it's too late to go back."

Anne fisted her hands. How dare he take that tone? How dare he talk to her like a kindly tutor, hesitant to teach his favorite pupil a harsh lesson?

"You raped my mother," she growled. "What could I learn that's worse?"

Kenton's face flushed and his chin jutted out as if she'd affronted him. "Very well. Here's the truth: I'd love to claim you, provide for you, offer the advantages you're entitled to. I always wanted that, but your mother refused it all. She preferred to save her reputation rather than see to your needs, so she claimed I assaulted her rather than admit our union was consensual. She's selfish and a liar."

Anne's internal fire died. Ice, so cold it hurt, spread inside. "That's not true."

"I assure you it is," Kenton said. "A gentleman doesn't accuse a respectable, unmarried woman of an amorous indiscretion, so I stayed silent. However, I had to refute the claim of rape to maintain my honor. I didn't ruin your mother's reputation. She did that on her own."

Blood surged in Anne's face, made her skin too tight, and tears pushed against the backs of her eyes. None of this was new, apart from him supposedly wanting to claim her, but hearing her father say it to her face was nauseating.

"You're claiming honor?" she hissed. "And a conscience? Don't you *dare* blame your lack of integrity on my mother."

Kenton took off his hat and raked gloved fingers through his hair: dark brown, without a trace of red. "I promised your mother I'd never approach you. I'd hoped, if you ever came to me, it would be warmer than this."

Anne stared at him. Had he truly imagined a joyful reunion with a long-lost daughter? Shock and disbelief surged through her veins, leaving her drunk with incredulity. If he'd truly wanted that, why had he never tried to catch her eye in church? Why had he left it all up to her? Why had he let his family be so cruel and dismissive to her? Was it truly to honor the request of her mother?

Her father's shoulders sagged, and he advanced a step. "The truth can be hard to face. Emma didn't accuse me until it became obvious she was with child. Claiming I forced her was an attempt to save her reputation."

"She was a frightened country girl! You were a married aristocrat, the most influential person in her world! Your assault made mincemeat of her. She didn't know what to do. She was afraid to tell her parents. She was ashamed—though she had no reason to be. Once she realized she was pregnant, she had no choice but to disclose what happened."

Kenton's head bent and slowly shook back-and-forth. Was he laughing? No. When his head lifted, Anne saw a man in pain. Face pale and lined, the corners of his mouth drooped. "I don't like denouncing your mother," he said, "and I'm not about to describe every detail, but she was a willing participant in our union. There. Was. No. Crime. At the time, I thought the most honorable course was to stay silent, and in deference to Emma I did. In hindsight, had I claimed you, I think the gossip would have died."

He was the best liar she'd ever met. Either that, or he believed it. Anne recalled her mum recounting the rape, describing how he'd laughed and complimented her spirit. Was it truly possible he thought their joining consensual?

She stared at the white mark still present on his left cheekbone. "When the lady's consenting, she doesn't leave a scar."

Kenton's hand flew to his cheek. He rubbed the mark, then his hand dropped and his eyes took on an intensity that made Anne avert her eyes. "That was an accident. Sometimes things happen in passion that are later regretted. You likely don't understand that. Or I hope you don't."

Her gaze flew back and reconnected with his. His restrained attitude, his calm reason filled her to bursting with resentment. She could barely hang on to her own control, barely suppress the urge to shout and scream, and her words were sharp, fast, heated. "Are you truly so arrogant you thought Mum's struggling was an act meant to appease her conscience?"

The possibility that he'd invented the explanation but also *believed* it made her stomach churn. Did he truly not feel guilt because he believed his own lies? And did that make him less of a monster or more?

His eyes closed, and a huge breath swept in and out of his lungs. He turned, passed his reins back over his gray's head, and mounted. Stared into the distance. "This exchange isn't beneficial to either of us. I'm sorry for you and your mother. I wish things were different." His gaze fell back upon Anne. "Other than my admission that I'm your father, was there something else you wanted?"

He *pitied* them? It seemed so. Thoughts, words, both were beyond Anne. He'd admitted he'd fathered her, as she'd always known he had, but he'd stuck to his position that Emma Albright was a willing participant in their encounter. Nothing had changed, really. Nothing except finally hearing it all from the man's own lips.

She shook her head. Kenton nodded curtly, heeled his horse and rode past her in the direction of the surgery.

Anne stared at Kenton's dust until her legs wilted like tulip stems deprived of water, and then with lurching steps she made her way to the low stone wall running along the road, and sat. A crazed-sounding laugh stuttered out. If possible, things were worse. She'd always known he lied, but now her usual certainty was riddled with a new angle of doubt. Had he told the lie so many times that he'd simply come to believe it true?

It didn't matter. Even if he'd spoken with the same authenticity that Rector Jennett read scriptures, even if her father honestly believed what he claimed, it didn't absolve him of rape. Her mother had fought him, and Kenton had pressed on. Hand cupping her midsection, Anne got to her feet like a stiff old woman and began the trek home. At the same time, she realized that Peter was wholly wrong. Talking to Kenton hadn't solved anything. It had only revived her pain and turned the world upside down.

~

Peter woke with a start in late afternoon light. A smiling Kenton faced him and the garden bench where he had nodded off just outside the surgery front door. A fine-looking gray stallion stood tethered to the hitching post.

His godfather walked forward. He and Peter clasped hands, a long, firm greeting that gave Peter a much-needed moment to come fully awake, and also giving time for Peter's initial surge of alarm to die. Anne wasn't here. She'd finished the day's work and gone home.

"You look well," Kenton said, sitting beside him on the bench. "What a relief. I wanted to forego my business and return straight-away, but Arthur assured me there was nothing I could do. And I ultimately see more orders for Pennyton stock from the connections made at Ascot than any other event. You were a constant worry, though, and several times I nearly gave it up."

Peter lifted his hand in a staying motion. "I was in good hands and

I'm mending. And I'm grateful you were saved the tedium of my indisposition. Now you can tell me the news from Ascot, which I've been anxious to hear. Did you take the new rail line?"

"Me and everyone else. Five trains a day ran each way. The Hunt Cup was phenomenal. I wish you could have seen it. A field of twenty-eight, so evenly weighted, descending the hill they looked like a line of charging cavalry. Near the finish, Muirland's Forbidden Fruit pulled away from the row and won by a neck."

Peter listened with only half an ear to words that would normally engross him. His heart was pounding, and he found certain questions couldn't wait. Questions that he knew would be almost impossible to speak.

His godfather leaned forward. "Enough about me. Tell me what you know about *you*. Have there been any further attacks? Have they found the shooter? And, why aren't you at Pennyton yet? I'll talk to Carter and get you moved tonight. No more excuses."

"Hold up," Peter managed. "We need to talk first."

Kenton raised open palms. "You needn't worry about endangering anyone at Pennyton. It's the safest place for you."

"This isn't about me." Peter paused, drew a breath for courage and then plunged ahead. "My concern is about what happened between you and Emma Albright all those years ago. I can't stay at Pennyton until I know."

Surprise flickered across Kenton's face, followed by a look of disbelief and pain. "You too? *You* think I attacked her?" A strong and athletic horseman, Peter's godfather shrank, his shoulders drawing in and his hands curling. "Peter, I…I'm shocked you'd even consider such a thing. Rumors and lies."

The disappointment in Kenton's eyes pressed upon Peter with the weight of the Bank of England's vault door, but he fought back, pushed past his guilt and fear. He had to be *certain*. This question had burned in him for weeks: What had happened on that day so long ago? How had the actions of this man, his godfather, a man who had been a distant shoulder to lean on, a steady stream of concerned advice and a constant tether to Peter's deceased father, affected Emma

Albright and her daughter, and possibly the entire village of Buttermere? Peter couldn't let his partiality blind him to the truth.

Kenton stood and paced. "Emma will answer for her lies when she stands before God," he said, his voice brimming with indignation. "As for this life, I don't know how she bears the shame."

Peter wondered the same thing. How *did* she? How did an inexperienced young woman find the strength to stand tall and make such a wicked accusation against the most powerful person in her community unless it was true? How did she face her church clergyman and lie for over twenty years? How did she tell her daughter her creation came from the damnable act of a depraved man unless she had righteousness supporting her? He *had* to know the truth.

"It was consensual, then? A love affair? Or did one of you seduce the other? I need to know exactly what happened."

Kenton stopped pacing, frowned, and drilled Peter with his eyes. But Peter stared back until Kenton shrugged and sniffed.

"It was a tumble in the grass. Nothing more. She'd been smiling and flirting for weeks. Shaking her tail like a bitch in heat."

Kenton crossed his arms, apparently finished, but it wasn't enough. Christ, this made Peter uncomfortable, but he had to press on. "The joining was consensual? She acted, and spoke, with desire? Always? Without variance? Without...encouragement?"

Peter's godfather rubbed the small white scar on his left cheek then resumed pacing; the grass in his path was now entirely flattened. "There was...some hesitation." His mouth puckered like he'd licked a lemon. "A complete pretense, and probably a scheme to lend credence to her later claims."

Peter was confused. "But you'd be the only one to know what passed between you. How would acting reluctant support any later allegation?"

"Well, perhaps it was to make herself feel better for abandoning her virtue. Or perhaps she wanted money all along, thought making me feel guilty would be advantageous. How am I to guess at her intentions?"

"She asked for money?" Peter asked.

Kenton slowed, rubbed his eyes, then stopped and faced him. "She would have, but I unintentionally insulted her when she confronted me with her pregnancy. Her pride is enormous." He shook his head. "And she's unstable. The accusation of rape followed. I offered money for the child even before she claimed I ravished her, but she refused. Foolish woman. I suppose, knowing her reputation was destroyed, she blamed me and wanted revenge. Hence the claim of rape. Withholding financial support was yet another evil act she could say I committed." He laughed, albeit harshly. "Or perhaps she thought I could be blackmailed into taking her as my mistress after all was said and done."

Peter could hardly process what he was hearing. His godfather believed Emma had refused his money as revenge? That seemed ridiculous. As ridiculous as refusing Kenton's money for any reason other than righteous fury.

"She was virgin?" he asked.

Kenton hesitated then gave a forceful exhale. "Yes."

Peter shook his head. "What you say makes no sense. I've met—"

"I don't know what was in the woman's mind, Peter. She was unreasonable, and I stopped trying to understand it all years ago."

"What about Anne, then? She's spent years desperately wanting you to love her. You've never even recognized her as your daughter. Not publicly."

Kenton grimaced. "She can thank her mother for that—for depriving her of the advantages even an illegitimate child of mine should possess." His brows snapped together. "You raking this up makes me question your judgment. I'd never have believed you capable of doubting me like this. Of thinking I could perpetrate something so vile. Perhaps I wasted my time on you, thinking I could be as good a friend to you as your father was to me. Thinking you were his son through and through. Your father would be ashamed at your lack of loyalty!"

What the hell? Peter's mind spun, and it took him a few moments to organize his thoughts and form words. His godfather was acting as if Peter were a faithful dog who'd unexpectedly turned savage and bitten. If only he knew how Peter loved Anne, he might understand—but Peter wasn't about to tell him. Not before he told Anne herself. Yet perhaps he could take a different tack.

"Miss Albright and I have become good friends," he explained. "Her mother helped care for me when I took a bad turn. I was stunned when I heard the stories. Wouldn't *you* investigate and find out the truth?"

Kenton grew an inch. "Not if the accusations were made against a man I loved and I knew better than such a thing. Not if that man had tried to be present for me at every opportunity since my father died. You apparently believe me capable of rape, as well as of telling the most immoral of lies!"

Irritation buzzed in Peter's chest like a swarm of midges. His godfather kept turning the focus to his perceived disloyalty, but Peter's first loyalty was to the truth. Even if it destroyed their relationship. With a look of disgust, Kenton shook his head. Which drew Peter's gaze to his godfather's small facial scar. "What did you mean, Emma showed 'some hesitation?'"

Kenton's eyes flashed. "It wasn't rape!" Fast and forceful, he swung his clenched fist downward in an ineffectual but violent motion, rocking forward, shaking, with his teeth clenched. "Understand?"

Good Lord. His godfather had turned into a red-faced, scowling, bull-necked monster. It was a side of the man Peter had never seen, and the vision brought an unwanted fear: Anne and her mother are right.

The front door of the surgery opened, and Edwin Carter strode out. "What's going on?" he barked, frowning.

Kenton barely glanced at him. He marched to his gray, tugged the reins free from the post and mounted. The stallion sidled and tossed its head but quieted as Kenton gained control, momentarily looking off into the distance. When that gaze refocused on Peter, there were lines in his godfather's forehead and a tired droop to his mouth, while he sat high in the saddle like a man falsely accused. He seemed to have regained his composure.

"Immediately upon arriving home, I headed here to see you. On my way, I encountered Anne Albright, and we had a… very sad and contentious exchange."

Anne had confronted Kenton? Impatience to know more swelled in Peter, and he could barely keep from bombarding the man with questions. But no, for now he'd heard enough from her father, and he'd also need to hear the details from her.

"I was upset, certainly not prepared for more of the same from you, Peter. I need some time, and we both need cooler heads. The day after tomorrow, Tuesday, I'll come back with my coach and transport you to Pennyton. We'll work through this there." Kenton's gaze flicked to Carter. "Away from naysayers and liars."

He didn't wait for Peter to reply, but put his heels to the gray and galloped away.

CHAPTER TWENTY-THREE

Mind whirling, heart pounding, Peter watched Kenton and horse recede. The thought that had burst into his head—that his godfather was guilty—suddenly seemed less certain. Kenton's furious, uncontrolled defense had sparked that reaction, but did one surprising loss of control prove the man capable of anything heinous, or had the man simply been overwhelmed by anger and hurt at what he viewed as Peter's unfair accusations? Wasn't it natural to be hurt by a godson's doubt?

Yes. Despite what had just happened, nothing was certain. Nothing was settled.

Carter stepped close and cleared his throat. Peter couldn't look at him. Bloody hell. The man was going to be full of questions he didn't want to answer. Not yet.

"I don't want to go to Pennyton Park," he said. "Shouldn't I stay here?"

"Funny thing," Carter answered, giving him an odd look. "I intended to tell you this evening. You're more or less ready for discharge."

"I'm fit?" Peter said.

"Not quite back to your normal strength and stamina, but you're coming along. You'll soon be regarding this time as a rather inconvenient and unpleasant interlude. I'd rather you wait a bit before traveling any real distance, just to be sure the fevers are gone for good, but I'm betting they are."

"Thank you," Peter said, though he felt only partially grateful for the diagnosis. "I doubt I would have survived without Miss Albright's and your care."

Carter nodded, then gave him another apprising look. "You don't have to go to Viscount Kenton's home. I can make arrangements for you to stay at The Fish Inn. You wouldn't be subjected to my surgery goings-on, and it's reasonable enough for a man of your means."

Peter stared at him. "I'm comfortable here. If it's all right with you, I'd rather not move. Not until I'm ready to move on for good."

Carter looked hesitant but then gave a nod. "All right. You're welcome to stay as long as I don't need your bed." He extended his arm. "How about a hand up? A nip of brandy wouldn't be out of order, either, while we wait for Mrs. Pettigrew to call us for supper."

The surgeon gave Peter a pull to help him to his feet, and they were shortly thereafter ensconced in a small area that was half sitting room, half office; Peter was surprised he'd never been inside it before. The surgeon packed his pipe with tobacco and disappeared out toward the kitchen, a moment later strolling back while drawing on the pipe's mouthpiece, holding a glowing coal to the bowl with ember tongs. Lighting ritual complete, he placed coal and tongs in a small bowl that appeared to be for tobacco ash, and moved to the corner cabinet. There, hefting a bottle of golden spirits and lifting his eyebrows, he asked without words if Peter cared to join him.

Peter nodded, and soon he had a short glass of brandy in hand. A quick taste caused a burst of heat like the celebratory flutter coursing through his blood at the pronouncement of his almost completed recovery.

Carter sipped his own brandy, settled into an upholstered chair at an angle to Peter's, and gave him a steady look. "It appears I'm missing some crucial information, like...you're acquainted with the viscount?"

"Yes, Mr. Carter," Peter admitted, trying to be as polite as possible.

"There's a lot I need to tell you, but I'd like to explain to Anne first. She should hear it before anyone else. If you could wait until tomorrow, I'd be grateful."

Silent, Carter gazed at him, his brow furrowed. "Is it something she's going to like hearing?"

Peter almost laughed. "No. She may never speak to me again." When Carter blinked and his gaze intensified, Peter muttered, "I suppose, given how you feel about her, you'll be glad of that."

"How I feel about her?" Carter echoed.

Peter nodded. The man hadn't commented on his use of Anne's first name, but that familiarity had to be another clue about Peter's feelings. He took another swallow of brandy and considered that, by tomorrow night, he might be wanting to drown himself in the spirit. "I saw from the first how well you thought of her, and of how comfortable you two are together."

Carter appeared to think that over. "I take it you..."

"Intend to make her my wife if she'll have me."

"Which perhaps she won't," the surgeon continued, "given your secret that I still don't know...?"

Peter couldn't bear to think of that possibility. Somehow, he had to make her understand. He hoped the good thing he had to say—that he loved her—would outweigh the devastating news that all this time he'd lied about who he was, and about the fact that the man she hated most in the world was his godfather.

Carter took the pipe from his mouth. "It's true I love Anne, but it's a brotherly sort of affection—as I told you before. Anne isn't the one I want to marry. It's Emma."

Well. Peter hadn't been expecting that.

"Emma Albright...?"

Of course Carter meant Anne's mother, but Peter didn't know what else to say. He didn't think the rousing cheer he felt like voicing would be appreciated. Not that Carter's lack of pursuing Anne would make much difference; he hadn't felt threatened by the man for some time now. Still, it was nice to think everyone could find love.

Carter's mouth thinned. "Yes. Any thoughts on the matter?"

Peter shook his head. "No. Just...have you told her how you feel? And if not, why not?"

"I've been afraid she sees me as a colleague and not a man. Worse, I'm nine years younger and was convinced that mattered." The surgeon paused. "I intimated my feelings early on. I invited her to dinner, sat beside her in church, and fixed her front steps. Offered to take her for a drive. She always seemed oblivious, as if it never occurred I might be trying to court her." He took another sip of brandy and rubbed his hand across his lower face, ruffling his mustache and beard. "But I've just had a hint that maybe she's interested after all. I've been working up the nerve to try again."

"Really?" Peter was happy for the man, even happier because perhaps he might win an ally in the struggle to claim Emma's daughter's hand. "How long have you had feelings for her?"

The surgeon gave a gusty exhale. "Since I settled here and opened my practice. Ten years."

Carter had been pining for Emma for ten years? "Good God, man. Why haven't you said something specific? Why dance around it?"

The surgeon flashed him a dark look. "We work together on occasion. I didn't want to do anything that might make her uncomfortable and affect our professional association." He placed the stem of his pipe in his mouth, drew upon it several times, frowned at the dead bowl, and set the pipe aside. He paused, then: "Especially because of her past. Do you...?"

"Yes. Anne told me."

Neither man spoke. The clock ticked. Peter and Carter both sipped their brandy.

"You understand, then," the surgeon said.

Peter did. He respected the man's solicitousness about Emma's feelings, too. However: "Ten years of patience and understanding is... impressive. To be frank, I don't know how you've managed."

Carter made a strange noise. When Peter glanced at him, he realized it was a laugh. Peter supposed there wasn't much else to do after waiting ten years to tell a woman you were interested in her.

"Take the risk and tell her how you feel," he said at last. "Especially if you think she may be interested. She might have turned that part of herself off for awhile, but perhaps she's ready to turn it back on. There are ways to be frank without threatening her peace of mind. You're a friend. Maybe you can show her a possibility she's never considered. And you can do it all while still being careful of her feelings. All you have to do is *listen*."

Carter appeared to be thinking. He pushed his spectacles up, rubbed his eyes, and let the lenses fall back into place. Then he nodded. "Of course you're right. I've wanted to tell her for some time. But I was afraid that my loving her would be a burden."

"Only if you force it on her," Peter said. "But isn't it fairer to both her and you to make decisions based on the truth?"

"It is," Carter said, his firm tone making it clear he'd made up his mind.

The truth. Peter found himself choking on the word. He and Anne deserved happiness, too, but the truth might stand in their way.

He didn't know the truth about anything except how he felt about her. He supposed that was as good a place to start as any.

CHAPTER TWENTY-FOUR

On her way to the surgery the next morning, Anne could barely contain herself. She wanted to *hurry*. Proud of finally facing her father, she was eager to tell Peter about the conversation. She'd told her mum, and Anne still felt buoyed from her mother's hug and the pride she'd seen in her mum's eyes at her daughter facing her fears.

Since it was Mrs. Pettigrew's half-day, and Edwin would be making home visits, she and Peter would have the place to themselves. Except, when Anne reached the surgery, Rector Jennett's gig sat outside. Anne sighed. Well, it wasn't the end of the world. He usually stayed about an hour; there'd still be plenty of time to talk before Edwin returned.

Entering through the back door, she hung her bonnet on the wall hook and headed toward the treatment and convalescent rooms. She stowed some bandage fabric in a cupboard and walked toward the convalescent room doorway. The men's voices grew louder as she neared.

"That's wonderful news, Peter!"

Her feet slowed. Mr. Jennett was using Peter's Christian name? That was odd. She'd never heard him do that before. The rector visited every day, and he and Peter had become friends, but not the kind of friends who used first names. Anne had known the rector for years, and he had never used her given name.

"I wish you could stay with Belinda and me, but I understand why you can't," Mr. Jennett went on. "Just don't ever let Mother find out. You know her philosophy. Family takes care of family, no matter what."

Anne froze looking through the doorway. Mr. Jennett sat in a highly casual pose in the convalescent room's cushioned chair, legs stretched out and feet crossed at the ankles. Her plans to tell Peter of the encounter with Kenton and of what they'd each said fell away. Only one thing filled her mind. "Who *are* you?"

Both the rector and Peter's gazes whipped to her. Mr. Jennett sat up. Peter stood, body tense and expression alarmed. Anne didn't know how he managed to move so smooth and fast, without a grimace or grunt.

"Anne."

Some part of her recognized the pleading in his tone, saw his unsupported arm raised in supplication, but she ignored both things. Her mind spun, trying to comprehend what the rector had said.

"Who are you?" she repeated, this time her voice an intense whisper, a betrayed and dying woman's last words.

Peter's arm dropped to his side and he grew taller. "I'm sorry, Anne, but I thought it would be safer to give a...a fictitious name when I came here. Someone was trying to kill me. Not just here, but before I arrived, back in London. I'm Peter Jennett, Viscount Easterbrook. Arthur and I...are cousins."

Cousins? Anne grabbed the door frame. Heat seared the backs of her eyes, burning cold filled her chest, and her flesh turned to granite. Peter started toward her, but she held up her hand and stayed him.

"I intended to tell you today."

He sounded earnest. Looked desperate. But he'd been lying all this time. Was she now supposed to trust he was telling the truth? Hadn't she even told him how much she hated liars? Told him when they were sharing what she thought was a moment of true intimacy. And *cousins*? Belinda was married to Peter's cousin?

"You intended to tell me the truth?" she managed to repeat. "Why ever was I included in your deception? You could have been honest from the beginning."

"I didn't know you. I didn't know whether you, or Carter, or Mrs. Pettigrew might tell my secret, in confidence, to someone else, and what would happen after that. I couldn't take the risk. My safety depended on tricking my assailant into thinking he'd shot the wrong man. And it worked. There have been no further attempts on my life."

Mr. Jennett got to his feet, face contrite. "My complicity helped perpetuate the lie. It's been a burden for both of us. I've prayed every day. I hope you can understand the necessity and forgive us, Miss Albright."

She'd worked with Mr. Jennett too many times, often comforting those grieving a departed loved one, to hold a grudge against him. He gave his all to God, his family, and his community. He would only have been listening to Peter and trying to see to his needs, so her hurt and escalating anger were for Peter, not the rector.

"I understand, Mr. Jennett," she said. "You were trapped by his lie."

"Would you leave us, Arthur?" Peter asked. "I'll talk to you tomorrow."

"Of course." Mr. Jennett was already halfway to the door. He paused to secure his hat upon his head, took a moment to look both Peter and Anne in the eye, then left. A small amount of the tension left with him.

"Please, sit down," Peter said.

Anne walked past him to the window, folded her arms, and stared without really seeing anything. A moment later, arms still folded, she spun and faced him. "I thought we were close," she blurted.

Oh, blast. That had spilled from her without a second's thought.

"We *are* close," he said, moving nearer. She shook her head, but he kept advancing. "We're more than just close." He was too near, an arm's length away. "I love you, Anne."

Her heart hitched. Had he really said that aloud? And, could he be as sincere as he looked and sounded?

White-hot, a sickening whirl of anger and pain wheeled through her shell of a body. "How can you say that you love me? You lied to me about who you are. Love is based on honesty, not deception. Whatever you think it is you feel, it's not love. Gracious God, your cousin is Belinda's husband! How could you hide *that* from me?"

His expression flickered, and she saw fear in his eyes.

"I hated lying to you. The time never seemed right to confess."

"You didn't trust me?"

"Of *course* I did."

"I shared everything," she reminded him. "My past, my feelings." It started as a trickle, but then other knowledge became a crashing, crushing avalanche of rocks. "But you know Mr. Jennet, so everything I told you...you already knew, didn't you?"

For an instant his face twisted like she'd plunged her scissors into his back, but a moment later she saw nothing but determination. His chest expanded and he said, "Anne. Please listen. Give me a chance to explain. The false identity gave me a degree of protection when I was otherwise unable to protect myself. Once I got to know you, I wanted to tell you everything but it was already too late. I knew that whenever you found out you'd be hurt and angry. I hoped the feelings we shared would prevail, but I was a coward and kept putting it off."

Another boulder crashed atop the pile of rocks on her chest. "Wait. Belinda knows all of this, too, doesn't she? All this time she's known."

Her half-sister had been in on the secret, and suddenly it seemed like collusion: Peter, the rector, Belinda, all sharing the secret, while Anne was left out, ignorant. Not just of who Peter was, but of the relationship they three shared. Had Peter discussed Anne with them? What a betrayal if he had. Even if he hadn't, Mr. Jennett had seen her reaction to learning the truth. He must realize Anne cared deeply for Peter. She bent her head, covered her face with her hands, and pressed her fingertips to her eyelids. The pain had grown too big to hold inside, and she didn't want him to see how much she hurt.

Peter came close. Even with her eyes covered, she knew he was there. Warm hands settled on her shoulders. Hands that seemed to hold her very, very fragile self together.

Hands. He'd taken his right arm from its sling.

"I love you," he repeated, low, deep, and steady. His hands squeezed gently. "I love you. Please don't let this come between us. It doesn't change anything. Not really. It doesn't change what's in our hearts."

Could he be right? What if she just…forgave him? Couldn't love transcend mistakes? He hadn't told her his true name, but hadn't he revealed his soul and spirit? Wasn't the inner man more important than his name? Hadn't he shown her as much when he talked about the deaths of his parents and fiancée? When he read to Michael and encouraged the boy's love of reading and learning?

He tugged her hands down and pulled her into his arms, and she let him. She rested her face on his chest, which somehow held the warm comfort of a bright sun on a blisteringly cold day. Nothing could feel better than being flush against him like this, his arms secure around her. Shouldn't it feel strange, or wrong, that the one responsible for her pain was also her source of solace? It didn't feel wrong. It felt right.

"I'm so glad you know now," Peter whispered into her ear. "I hated the deception, and I've lived in dread of you finding out. I feared you'd despise me."

"Are you really a viscount?" Anne whispered, the reality washing over her. It was the same detested title her father possessed. Since childhood she'd associated it with arrogance and privilege and cruelty.

Peter's arms tightened and he swayed, rocking her. "Yes."

They both fell silent. Anne concentrated on his solid heat, on his fingers sliding up and down her spine. Then he leaned away, creating a small space between them.

"Anne."

She didn't respond. He gave her a little jostle, and she opened her eyes. Could she trust him now? Everything about him seemed open. She took her time, probing his gaze and finding truth and longing and a pledge. Tension built behind her heart and squeezed into her throat.

She wanted to believe him. *Yearned* to trust him. But was she deceiving herself, seeing things that weren't real?

He'd lied for a reason. She should learn what that was.

"Someone's trying to kill you. Who? Why?"

"I wish I knew. I came here intending to hide away with Arthur for a time. When I was shot, I immediately became fearful of endangering his family and so gave a false name in the hope it would mislead the gunman, whom I assumed followed me from London. But I'm not entirely sure of anything. The constable has known the circumstances since the beginning, and I hired his son Owen to go to North Yorkshire and investigate one of my businesses—a colliery I had to close. He thinks he found the man, but that man disappeared." Peter paused. "The shooting was the third near-death experience I've had in the past six months. I expected more."

A dagger of ice slid through Anne's heart. "You're still in danger, then?"

"No." Peter shook his head. "At least, I don't think so. The miners are working again, and the colliery will soon be back up and running." He released a gusty sigh. "I really did mean to tell you everything today. I'm sorry you found out the way you did."

Anne stared at him. Peter had arrived gravely injured. Helpless and afraid. Insensible. He'd lied hoping to protect himself. He'd claimed he intended to tell her the truth today, and his gaze held love. Worry and regret, too, but most of all, love. Yes, she believed him. Believed his words, and even more, what she saw in his eyes.

She leaned in, brushing her lips against his. Soft and easy, he responded; his mouth coaxed, invited. Tingles danced along the back of Anne's neck, across her shoulders, and down her arms. The drawing sensation focused in her feminine parts was so strong she might have been iron and Peter a lodestone. Her body wanted his, yes. Her mind wanted to ignore warnings and questions and fears. Her *soul* wanted—

He kissed her, and the tightness in her chest unfolded and became the fragile wings of a butterfly. Wings that opened. A sense of rightness filled her: She belonged here in Peter's arms. She'd never been so certain of anything.

They kissed again and again, lips caressing, tongues stroking, and the pulling sensation in her core grew stronger and stronger. She palmed his back and pressed against him, pushing into his heat and tension. This, then, was carnal desire. Shouldn't she be resisting? Not a single part of her wished anything but to follow through and sample the full banquet of love's joys. But where would that lead? What was she doing?

Peter stopped kissing her but then started again. Once, twice, three times. "Anne." His eyes glinted, and his thumb brushed her lower lip. "I'm not sure we're ready. Not right now, not when someone's tried to kill me and I'm still something of an invalid. All I know for certain is nothing could be better, more right, than being with you always. I want that more than I've ever wanted anything. Please, will you marry me?"

Be his wife? Bear his children, spend all her days beside him? Exhilaration buzzed under her skin and swirled in her belly. This was everything she'd ever wished. Her life would know love—more love than she'd ever dreamed.

Except, it wasn't as easy as that.

"It's not that simple," Anne pointed out. "I'd need to become your *viscountess*. I can't even imagine such a thing." She had no idea of what she'd be required to do, or how to act. Might he even be criticized for wedding her?

"You're not the usual viscountess, but you'll be an exquisite one," he assured her. Stroking her arm, elbow to wrist, he took her hand. "I'm not concerned with your filling the usual role. I want the woman who's a match for the man I am *here*." He pressed her hand to his heart, and tingles chased over her arms. "My parents were lucky enough to find love, and I want the same. I *deserve* the same. You're the right woman, and I only worry I'm not good enough for you. But, if you'll have me, I pledge to love you and stand beside you for all our days."

She stared into his eyes, trying to process all he was saying. He drew her to the bed and pulled her down to sit beside him.

"I've lain in this bed and listened, my admiration growing with each passing day. You amaze me, Anne Albright. You've comforted and protected, been smart and brave and tenacious. And most of all, you make people's lives better. I'll try my best to be a man worthy of you. I promise."

Anne wanted to believe it all and surrender to this dream, but she couldn't quite imagine them together. Her initial joy drained away; despair pinched her heart. He'd nearly died, and facing mortality changed a person—but not always for good. His judgment might be clouded at the moment, and where would they be a year from now? Very far from the Lake District, in a London townhouse or at the seat of the Viscounts Easterbrook. Places very different than Buttermere village.

"You admire my fine qualities and I admire yours," she conceded.

"Mine?" he said, his eyebrows shooting up. "I've done nothing but lie in bed. And lie to you."

She shook her head. "Not just that. You've pushed yourself, refused to give up, and even in pain retained your humor and kindness. You've looked out for those other than yourself. So, yes," she said, staring into his eyes and wishing things were different, "we've mutual esteem and friendship and desire, but..."

How to make him understand? She paused, took a breath, gathered her courage. "What about the rest of the world? You're an aristocrat. You may discount our different statuses, but I don't. I'm illegitimate, Peter. A *nurse*. I'd never fit into your world."

He gave a slow nod, clearly listening. "To be honest, some of our contentment will depend on you—on how you come to terms with the opposition we encounter. Because you're right, not all will accept you. Please believe this: I don't care about the opinions of those too short-sighted, prejudiced, and uncharitable to accept you. There are plenty who will, and I think some of the others we'll convert. The world is changing, and the aristocratic world is being forced along. Some, like me, are enjoying and contributing to the change."

She leaned closer and squeezed his arm. "Even if I thought there was a chance I'd be accepted, it's about more than what I am. It's *who* I am. If I couldn't nurse, part of me would disappear."

He placed his hand atop hers. "We'll find a way to use your skills, and make you fit into my blue-blooded world, too."

Could that be true? Florence Nightingale had been a lady from a noteworthy family and she'd found a way to nurse. She'd set her mind to a goal and made it happen. Anne supposed the famous nurse believed a woman could do anything she set her mind to.

Peter ran his hands up her arms and rested them on her shoulders. His thumbs circled her clavicle bones. "So much analysis. There's one thing that matters more than anything else. *Do you love me?*"

She did. Could she forgive his deception? Yes. He had given a false identity for good reason, and a different name didn't change the man he was. Could she become a viscountess? Possess the same hated title her father held? She'd be the man's social equal. That thought brought a stab of panic.

Peter cupped her jaw with his palms and gave her a strong kiss. "Marry me."

Her throat tight, her heart bursting, her answer came out in a husky murmur. "Yes.

CHAPTER TWENTY-FIVE

"I love you," Anne said, and she put her fullness of feeling into the words. She hadn't known a kiss could be at once happy and passionate, but Peter gathered her to him, and wherever their skin touched a current of delight and desire flowed. Yes, she belonged in Peter's strong arms, pressed to his chest. She felt his hunger as he kissed her, and certainty settled deep inside.

His lips trailed across her cheek, and his nose nuzzled her temple. "Thank you for understanding. I've been afraid you wouldn't be able to accept it all. Now that you know, there's so much more I need to say, to explain."

"Tell me later." Anne wrapped her arms around his neck.

But...he pulled back. Enough that she had to loosen her arms to see his eyes, and his expression seemed to convey a warning that, for just an instant, made her heart stutter. Because, instead of a reflection of her joy, she glimpsed apprehension and worry and determination.

"I need to tell you now. It's important. I—"

"Please. I don't want to hear anything that might spoil this moment." With her finger she smoothed the crease between his brows. Did he intend to qualify their love? Compare it to what he'd felt for Louisa? That was the only conversation she feared and didn't want, and what else would he consider so important right now? "You told me everything I need to know. Right now, I want to think about how marvelous our future will be. Is that selfish of me? I spent my life wondering if I'd ever fall in love, and if I did, what it would feel like, and already it's better than I imagined."

Happiness came into his expression, and some of the worry went away. Her worry receded, too. She yearned to be a bit forward, to experience more, and her cheeks burned. Did she dare ask? Would he find it offensive? But, no. She trusted him.

"I'd be far more persuadable about listening after more…kisses." And for the second time she gathered her courage and touched her lips to his.

Wondrous.

Another kiss followed. And another. Kiss after kiss after long, slow, astounding kiss. The bundle of nerves in her stomach loosened and melted into a warm pool. As one, she and Peter lay back on the bed. He stretched half atop her, half alongside, and she wanted to never move. His hands—strong, masculine hands—slid over her back and waist and breasts. Beneath the unyielding obstruction of her corset and too many clothes, her skin warmed and tingled. His caresses seemed to grant permission for her to touch and embrace him, and she slid her hands up his chest and over his back and waist and even lower, over his bum. Her nursing work had given her more understanding of male anatomy than other unmarried women, but studies and nursing service had never made her heart fill her chest, nor made her marvel. She'd never felt like this, never in her whole life, so full to bursting yet needing more. She'd become a different woman in his arms: a woman loved.

But a moment later his hands stilled and he drew away, his eyes and mouth tight like a man in pain, and he shook his head as if shaking off sleep. "We have to stop. Or in a few minutes I'll be stripping off your clothes."

She didn't want to stop. She didn't think he did, either. But he was an honorable man and wouldn't be removing her clothing or pulling up her skirts until after they were wed. She, more than most, knew life was short and took unexpected and sometimes tragic turns. She'd spent her life wondering and searching for this, for Peter, and now the desire to experience the fullness of his love was overpowering.

He moved a little farther away. "I must finish explaining."

She'd already listened and reasoned and accepted, and the thought of doing more of that, when her entire being was vibrating with want, she couldn't fathom. Especially if his explaining had to do with Louisa. Or even if it was about something else. She didn't want to let this feeling go.

She gripped his arm. Nerves bunched the pit of her stomach. All her life she'd been careful to never show even a hint of impropriety. But, then, she'd never experienced this kind of compulsion and certainty. And this was Peter. He would understand.

She took a deep, steadying breath. "First tell me… Can we marry soon?"

"As soon as possible. Arthur can perform the ceremony."

His straightforward, honest gaze demolished the last, lingering bit of her reticence. "Then don't make me wait."

Peter laughed—or coughed, she couldn't tell which—and clamped her waist as if determined not to move closer. "We should wait until we're joined as man and wife."

Yes. Joined, Anne agreed. As man and wife. For suddenly she knew what they must do.

"You can tell me everything tomorrow," she promised. For a moment the magnitude of what she was doing overwhelmed her, but she filled her lungs and, along with the air, peace spread through her chest. "But today—now—we can make our pledge to God." She kissed Peter, lingering a long moment. "Join our souls and our bodies. Please. I've never shared myself, never done more than exchange a kiss or two, but I know *this* is the way love is supposed to feel. This is not wicked or shameful or shocking, it's love and joy prevailing the way God intended."

Love radiated from Peter's face, spilled from his eyes, and relief surged in Anne's brain and cascaded through every cell. She knew behind his open expression of love, banked passion simmered. Never before had she felt true passion, but she recognized it in both Peter and herself.

Then he closed his eyes. His expression of delight disappeared like a room going dark, and when his eyes opened she saw hard determination. It made her heart slow, her blood go cold, and her relief die. He was going to refuse.

"I've more experience than you, but none of it matters because I've never felt anything like this. It's because of how I love you that I want our union to be perfect. I want us both to be free of the past, saying our vows with open minds and open hearts. No shadows."

"*Trust me,* then," she begged. "Trust our love, and don't make me wait. Because this is right. Nothing has ever felt so right. I promise you, I'll have no regrets."

Again he started to speak, but she stopped him, pressing her fingers against his lips. She seemed to wait forever. Then he took her hand, kissed her fingertips, and nodded. *Oh, thank God.* She laid her hand over his heart. Breathed in rhythm to the rise and fall of his chest. And felt one with him.

"Then let us speak our vows." She took a deep breath. "Peter Jennett, I promise to stay beside you through all the days and nights of our lives. With all the resolve of my heart, I bind my life to yours. I pledge my love and loyalty and fidelity."

His fingers tightened upon her other hand, and he sighed. "I pledge myself to you, Anne Albright. Everything I have to give is yours: all I own and all I am. I promise to be faithful, to protect you and love you always."

Anne's eyes filled with tears. She shifted her hand so she and Peter were palm-to-palm, slid her fingers between his, and joined their hands. Hands, hearts, lives—they were connected as surely as if they'd spoken their vows in St. James before Mr. Jennett.

She met his advancing lips and her heart soared like a kite in a fresh wind. His mouth turned that wind into a storm. She pressed against him but encountered clothing, too much clothing: skirts and petticoats and corset and long-sleeved bodice and buttons marching down that bodice.

She released his hand and pushed a button through its buttonhole. This time, he didn't object. He looked at her intently for a moment then rolled away, off the bed, and strode to the door. She worked more buttons as he closed and locked it. Then he drew the curtains. He re-crossed the room and helped as she pulled her arms from her bodice sleeves; she released her corset, and he worked his shirt off without lifting his right arm. She untied skirts and petticoats, and he unlaced and removed her boots.

At last they lay together again, she in chemise and stockings, he in drawers and undershirt. They might as well have been naked, for the two layers of cotton that separated them were soft and thin and amounted to nothing. Together, their bodies generated a heat to rival the hottest summer day, and Anne's skin became damp and sensitive and attuned to the smallest contact.

She kissed Peter's mouth, nerves drawing tight while her fingers traced muscular bulges and bony ridges. Delight made her explore further, caressing hard masculine slopes and swells and making his breathing jerk.

His hands on her breasts almost made her cry out. She'd lost control of her body. The flesh between her legs, her womb, and her breasts seemed to strain for his touch. He rubbed the tips of her breasts, her nipples contracted, and between her legs everything feminine clenched. She gasped.

He kissed her, a kiss of power and intensity, a kiss that revealed a hunger that matched her all-consuming desire. His hands went to *that* place, and when he touched her, she moaned. He rubbed and it felt so amazing it sent frissons chasing over her hot skin and she wanted... wanted...wanted...

Her hips lifted. His finger slid inside her, and there was more tightening and more frissons and more...more...

He pressed his pelvis against hers and rubbed his hardness over that most sensitive part of her. She squeezed her hand between them, slid it inside his drawers, and when she touched his rigid cock, harder and larger than she'd imagined a man could be, he made room for her stroking. He groaned, guided her fingers, and her confidence grew. More powerful kisses that made desire burn through her body, made her want him—his cock—there. Inside her.

She pushed his drawers off his hips and he shifted over her. The head of his cock nudged at her entrance and she thought she might die with the wanting. He was breathing like he couldn't get enough air, and suddenly she knew he was moving slowly to avoid hurting her. She pulled his hips toward her and lifted her pelvis, and he finally thrust into her with a deep, guttural groan.

It pinched sharper and harder than she'd expected, but the pain lasted only seconds before beginning to ease. He moved, and she locked her legs around him.

"I didn't know," he murmured, slowly withdrawing and advancing.

"Didn't know?"

"Didn't know it could feel like this."

He sounded happy and thankful and amazed. She understood. Each time he moved, it was like an ocean wave moving through her, sweeping in and out, each swell deeper and stronger. Each carried her closer to the crest. It was a physical feeling, but even deeper and stronger was love.

The lingering discomfort ebbed. Anne swept higher, higher, impossibly high. Then, with a final surge, the wave broke. Moments later Peter went rigid and she heard his deep sound of satisfaction and release. She drifted in timeless wonder. They clung together, sweating and breathing hard. She'd been wrung, and splayed, and she felt glorious.

Peter twisted down alongside her, and they lay facing each other. He smoothed a lock of mussed hair away from her face, then curled his hand around the back of her neck. She cupped his bearded jaw, searching his eyes. The gray rim encircling the blue was difficult to see unless she was very close, but she intended to see it often now. She'd first noticed it when he'd arrived unconscious, and she opened his eyelids to check his pupils. Then she'd been detached, a nurse examining a patient. Now she saw the eyes of the man she loved, brimming with feeling for her.

"I'm so very happy," Peter said. He rubbed his thumb across her lower lip and gave her a tender kiss. "You are sunshine."

Anne smiled. "If I am, it's because of you."

CHAPTER TWENTY-SIX

Hours later, Peter continued to smile. Until today, the greatest euphoria he had ever felt was standing on the Grossglockner summit. Today he walked on clouds far above that towering peak. Anne loved him.

After their lovemaking, while Anne dressed, she'd quickly told him about her encounter with Kenton. "He's a disturbed man. I'm so glad Mum insisted we have nothing to do with him." Hurrying to be ready for the late morning patients, she hadn't said more. Neither had Peter. Mrs. Pettigrew arrived and soon after served luncheon, which they all ate together. Afterwards Peter tried to read one of his architecture books, but he kept catching himself listening for Anne's voice and grinning like a fool.

The lovely day proceeded, enhanced by a stolen kiss once when they were alone. Carter arrived back just as Peter was reluctantly seeing Anne off toward home. After she left, he tried reading again, but he just ended up watching his spider. The web was now of a size that made Mrs. Pettigrew shake her head and tsk-tsk every time she entered the room, but she continued to leave his rather strange entertainment unharmed. Before he left the surgery, he'd transfer the insect to the hydrangea bush, he decided. He gave a nod of thanks to the spider, who apparently was making a meal of the pesky fly that had annoyed him earlier.

That evening, the meal Mrs. Pettigrew served was a simple one, but Peter found the repast as enjoyable as any he'd ever eaten. Apparently love enhanced the flavor of food.

Finished, Carter leaned back and gave Peter a questioning look. "Given that you're the picture of happiness, I hardly need ask," the surgeon said, "but did you have your talk with Anne? Everything all right between you?"

"More than all right. We're betrothed. Although I'd like to make sure her mother has no objections." They'd spoken vows. In Peter's eyes—and in God's eyes as well, he believed—they were already wed. Peter wasn't sharing that with Carter, though. The surgeon would draw the likely—and accurate—conclusion that they'd consummated their union.

Carter's eyebrows shot up, and he looked more irritated than pleased. That surprised Peter, but the surgeon's next words clarified the issue.

"Betrothed? Congratulations. So you're planning on stealing my nurse away, are you?"

Peter gave a nod. "Arthur Jennett is my cousin. I intend for him to perform the ceremony before I leave, so Anne can accompany me. I know she'll hate leaving you in the lurch, but I'd like us to depart as soon as you think I'm able."

Carter seemed to consider. "Perhaps her mother can help out here. I assume this means you're ready to tell me your secrets—and your relationship to Mr. Jennett isn't the only detail you've withheld. I hope I'll be just as happy for Anne once I hear what you have to say."

Peter did too. It was time to explain who he was. "I'm Viscount Easterbrook. That shooting was intentional, and I hoped a false name would divert my assailant. It appeared to do the trick."

With a long whistle, Carter removed his spectacles and polished the lenses, shaking his head. He secured the eyewear back on his face. "No question but she loves you if she's agreed to become a viscountess."

"I had to convince her," Peter admitted with a grin. "I can't imagine any other woman even pausing for an instant at the opportunity to become an aristocrat."

Carter nodded, staring at him, and Peter recalled that somehow he'd never explained his connection to Kenton. He would, though, first thing tomorrow. Until Anne knew, Peter would withhold that part of his history from Carter.

"I suppose Constable Weaver knows? The shooter's been apprehended?"

"Not apprehended, but I think we've identified him, and I have reason to believe the danger is past. Owen Weaver's recent journey was on my behalf."

Carter nodded. "Young Weaver returned a very different man than when he left, in a good way. I've seen him when he drops by—to make reports to you, I imagine." The surgeon stood, left the room, and returned with the previous night's now familiar bottle of brandy, saying, "I believe a celebratory dram is in order." Drinks poured, he then made a toast to "The health and happiness of you and Anne."

Peter sipped and marveled at all the joy to come. He and Anne had only just declared their love, and he'd never been so happy.

In bed, he found himself surrounded by Anne's fragrance. He turned his head to the pillow, inhaled a slow pull of the rose scent, and pictured her lying beside him after their lovemaking. He'd turned his back while she washed and dressed but watched when she repaired her hair. He hadn't stopped grinning all day. Completely relaxed, he closed his eyes. It wouldn't be long now, and he'd replace memories and this lingering fragrance with Anne herself.

A few hours later, Peter was awakened in darkness by a pounding on the surgery door and a man's distressed voice telling Carter that Emma Albright needed him fast. Peter listened to Carter leave, and then he let his mind drift back toward sleep.

Sometime later he awakened again, the room still dark, but instead of drifting in drowsy comfort, his brain flashed fully awake. Nearly silent, quick, shallow breathing and a soft, furtive tread warned him.

Someone was here. *Close.* Not Carter, not Anne. Someone who shouldn't be here.

Peter lunged toward the knees of the dim figure that appeared beside his bed, but something slammed into his left upper arm and it exploded with pain. He dove away, hit the floor, and scrambled up next to the little table that held his glass of water. Fury gave him strength to ignore the devil-pain that overwhelmed and paralyzed his arm, and Peter grabbed the table leg and swung the entire thing toward the attacking figure's head. The water glass went flying and shattered somewhere. The man ducked and turned, and the table broke across his upper back.

A man of a similar height and size as Peter. Was he holding a weapon? A pistol?

Get close. Hurt him.

Before Peter could act, a fist hit his stomach and drove the air from his lungs. Bent over, he staggered, trying desperately to breathe. *Move, damn it! He's going to kill you!*

He seized a sharp, tiny breath and plowed his head into his assailant's hard belly. They both went down, his enemy with a curse. Peter landed hard, and stars filled his vision. His arm throbbed and he gasped for air.

The small amount of moonlight spilling in the window wasn't enough to reveal anything but his assailant's dark shape getting to his hands and knees. What was he doing, scrabbling about on the floor? *Searching for his weapon. I have to get it first.* On his back, Peter placed himself at a right angle to his assailant, lifted his legs and slammed his feet into the thug's side. The man sprawled, but soon after began to move. He got to his feet, shuffled, grunted, then—

The toe of a boot. Fire exploded in Peter's side. *Ohhhhh, Jesus.*

"What the—?" Carter's voice from the doorway.

Peter's assailant ran—right through Carter and...another person? A woman gave a startled shriek, and Peter heard bodies hit the floor. He clutched his side and strained to hear more, and he got sounds of a tussle: scrabbling, grunts, fists striking flesh, furniture crashing—

possibly chairs along the waiting room wall—and another feminine cry. Boots ran toward the front door and then, nothing.

"Emma?" Carter's terse voice.

"I'm all right," Emma Albright said, her voice high-pitched and uncertain.

Sounds followed of Carter giving chase, trailing the fleeing ruffian out the door. Slowly, slowly, slowly, Peter sat up. In the hallway, light dispelled the darkness, and Anne's mother appeared carrying a lantern. She knelt beside him.

"Where are you hurt?"

"My left arm and ribs," Peter said through gritted teeth, cradling his injured arm against his side. "I think they're broken."

Emma patted his knee. "I'm sorry. Let's make your arm more comfortable before you move again."

His sling, which he'd all but stopped using, lay on the floor. The previous weeks it had supported his right arm and kept his shoulder blade immobile as it healed. Now Emma put his left arm inside the wide loop of silk and knotted the ends behind his neck.

"Is that better?"

He nodded, frustrated. "Yes."

"Can you get up? I'll help," Emma said.

"No, let me," Carter interjected, limping into the room. He glanced at Peter but took Emma's arm and helped her stand. "Are you all right, Emma?"

"A little bruised," she admitted, rubbing her hip. "But I'm fine. What about you? You took the brunt of the fall, trying to keep me safe. How badly are you hurt?"

"My spectacles are lost out there in the dark," Carter said in an aggrieved tone. He rubbed the bridge of his nose, which was red and already swelling.

"You're limping," Emma noted crossly.

Carter gazed at Peter. "He got away. I never even got a look at him. He had his face covered, and a horse hidden behind the house."

"I'm lucky you came home when you did," Peter said. "I'm pretty sure my upper arm's broken, and my ribs on the left hurt like—" There was a lady present, he remembered. "The blazes."

Carter glanced at Emma, then frowned at Peter. "It was late when we finished. I was escorting Mrs. Albright home. On our way past we decided...to restock a few of the supplies she used tonight."

Both Carter and Emma blushed, and in spite of his pain Peter had to lower his head in order not to smile. Most would doubt such a middle-of-the-night excuse, and assume them engaged in risqué conduct. Peter believed them, though. He wished, for both their sakes, he *had* caught them *in flagrante delicto.*

The surgeon crouched beside Peter and checked the pulse in his throbbing arm. "Let's get you to bed, and I'll check your injuries."

Peter took a deep breath, and with Carter's assistance, stood. "Queen Victoria's cat, but that hurts." He blindly obeyed the limping surgeon, and was soon reclining on his bed with great relief.

Emma stepped out, returning with a small knife for Carter, and a burning spill. She lit the lamp atop the chest of drawers, blew out the spill and tossed it into Peter's chamber basin. Then she picked up the first lamp she'd brought in, and left the room.

Carter cut and tore the shoulder seam of Peter's nightshirt and examined his arm. "It's fractured, all right," he said. With a sigh he sat on the edge of the bed.

"You're hurt," Peter said.

"Wrenched my ankle when I fell," he said in a dismissive tone, "and I didn't do myself any favors when I ran on it. What about your other injuries?"

"He kicked me in the ribs, but I don't think they're broken. Just bruised." He hoped.

Carter raised Peter's nightshirt and palpated his left ribcage. Sharp pain tore through Peter's chest. He couldn't hold back the moan.

"Probably cracked," Carter said, straightening. "At least your broken humerus doesn't look displaced. I'll splint the fracture, and you're to keep your arm in the sling and not use it. Luckily your scapula is pretty well healed. You can use your right hand."

Emma returned toting crutches and held something out for Carter. His spectacles.

"I found them," she said. "They're not damaged."

Carter stood, stuck the crutches under his arms, and put the spectacles on. He grinned. "Thank you."

"I'll wrap your ankle and give Mr. Matthews laudanum," Emma said. "You too, if you need it, and then I'll fetch the constable."

Her calling him Matthews made Peter realize she didn't yet know his real name.

"This attack was an attempt to murder me," he said. "My name is Peter Jennett. I'm Viscount Easterbrook, Rector Jennett's cousin. I explained everything to Anne yesterday."

Except, he *hadn't* told Anne everything. Looking at Emma Albright reminded him he'd wanted to reveal all, but he hadn't. He'd listened to Anne when she asked him to wait, telling himself she'd had enough shocks for the day. She'd learned who he was, about his relationship to Arthur and Belinda, and that someone wanted him dead. The idea of waiting a few hours, letting her grow accustomed to those truths before hitting her with the biggest shock of all—his connection to her father—seemed a sensible idea. Now the decision to wait seemed bad. Stupid. Disastrous.

Emma's wide-eyed, slack-mouthed reaction to his confession lasted only a moment, then she grimaced. "I was called out before Anne got home, so I didn't see her. How did she take the news?"

"Once we talked, she understood. She agreed to be my wife. I hope you'll wish us happy."

The smile that broke across his future mother-in-law's face made a fountain of relief surge high within Peter. She didn't approach, though, instead whirling toward Carter.

"Isn't it wonderful?" she exclaimed, throwing her arms around the surgeon. Then, one long, exuberant hug later, she backed out of his arms. "Forgive me," she said, laughing, her color high. Her star-bright eyes flashed to Peter and she stepped forward. They clasped hands, and he realized she was crying tears of joy. "It's just that I'm so happy. I knew she thought you were special."

Peter just smiled. Emma's gaze flicked back to Carter, and her color heightened again. She spun and stepped toward the door. "Shall we take care of your ankle?"

Carter crutched after Emma into the treatment room. Peter closed his eyes and listened with half an ear as Emma asked Carter to remove his shoe. Then a chill skated over Peter's flesh. Someone was still after him. John Monroe? If not Monroe, then who? Owen Weaver was due to report in soon, and the two of them would have to figure this out.

Meanwhile, remaining at the surgery was no longer feasible. His presence would endanger all these good people. He didn't want to go to Pennyton Park, but Kenton's estate, surrounded by acres of parkland, with servants inside and out, was the safest choice.

Out of sight, Carter's voice drifted through the open door.

"Please, don't be embarrassed, Emma. The past several years, nothing has felt as good as your arms around me tonight."

Peter knew he should quietly hum or whistle so as not to violate their privacy. Instead, he tilted his head and listened with hope.

"Edwin."

Anne's mother sounded a little shocked and a lot unsure, but she'd used Carter's given name, which was encouraging.

"I'm...older."

"Not in any way that matters," Carter said.

"My reputation—"

"Doesn't matter to me," he said, cutting her off. "Nothing would make me prouder than to escort you to Sunday service and show the entire parish how highly I regard you."

A rustle of clothing and faint shuffle of shoes. A soft sound of surprise from Emma. Peter imagined Carter had stepped close, perhaps even pulling her into his arms.

"I've been in love with you for years," Carter said, so low Peter barely heard him. "Won't you give me a chance?"

A long silence followed, which seemed a very satisfactory answer.

CHAPTER TWENTY-SEVEN

The next morning, the anticipation of seeing Peter almost had Anne dancing through the surgery front door. But when she entered, she came face-to-face with Constable Weaver, Owen Weaver, and Edwin, who was supported by crutches. The room was full of male tension. Something was wrong.

"Good morning, Miss Albright," Constable Weaver said. "Lord Easterbrook was attacked last night."

She mentally jolted at his use of Peter's title. Evidently they all knew who he was.

"His left humerus is fractured and a couple ribs cracked or bruised," Edwin said. "The constable found a hammer that was knocked under the bed during the scuffle."

"Scuffle?" *Hammer*? Anne's heart lurched, then beat as though the organ was trying to batter its way through her ribs. "Someone broke his arm with a *hammer*?" She pressed her hand to her chest.

"The ruffian escaped," Constable Weaver said, frowning. "For now," he added, low and growly. "Owen will be providing Lord Easterbrook with protection until he's settled elsewhere."

She started toward Peter's room, then paused and looked at

Edwin's leg. His shoe was off. A wrap extended above the top of his sock. "You were injured?"

"I was called to help your mother last night, and we didn't finish until very late. When I came in, the assailant and Peter were fighting."

"Mum was still sleeping this morning. I didn't wake her."

"The thug ran, and I chased him. Bad luck, I wrenched my ankle. It's swollen and painful but not broken. This morning I can't put weight on it. You'll need to make all the home visits for a week or so."

"Peter's all right?"

"A simple break. Set and splinted. His ribs are wrapped."

She nodded and went through to Peter. Her heart turned over when she saw how pale he was, semi-propped up, lying against his pillows. A heavy ache spread through her chest. She wanted to wrap her arms around him and hug him close.

He sighed. "Thank God. You're here." He held out his right hand, and she hurried to the far side of the bed to take it. As Edwin had said, a leather splint, extending to the height of his armpit, had been tightly laced around his upper left arm. The splint, and the sling the arm rested in, would keep the arm immobile.

"Are you all right?" Her voice came out a little jagged. She swallowed.

"I'm fine, but I need to tell you something."

"Edwin explained. Did you see the man who attacked you?"

"It was too dark to make out much."

"There was a nosy stranger here last week. Remember? Could it have been him?"

"It's possible," Peter said. "Please. Sit down. I need to talk to you."

He seemed different than how she'd expect to find him. Impatient. Even nervous. She heard a carriage and horses, and Peter glanced toward the window. He squeezed her hand and gave her a long, pained look.

"That's Kenton," he said.

"How do you know?" Was Kenton somehow involved in Peter's attack?

"I can't stay here any longer. The man from last night could return.

Others, like you, Edwin, or Mrs. Pettigrew, could be placed in danger. Likewise, I can't stay at Arthur's or the inn. I'm going to Pennyton Park."

What? A giant pin stabbed through Anne's center. "Pennyton Park. Are you joking?" Why would he go there? It wasn't possible.

Then her father strode in, with Edwin, Constable Weaver, and Owen Weaver filing in behind him. Anne's body turned to rock.

Kenton went straight to Peter, giving her and Peter's joined hands a brief glance. She jerked her hand free and stepped back. Her spine hit the wall.

"You should have been at the Park from the beginning," Kenton said to Peter. "It's where you belong, son."

The world—*her* world—was spinning, tipping, tearing, becoming a place she didn't know. Anne had been thrown into a locale inhabited by apparitions who looked identical but were completely different than the real people she knew. She looked at Peter, silently begging him to explain and make sense of this craziness.

"Viscount Kenton is my godfather, Anne. I've known him all my life. I wanted to tell you—"

Anne's hands flew up, as if she could stop the words. *No. It can't be.* Her mouth worked but nothing came out. Her mind grappled, tried to make sense, tried to comprehend. Then understanding struck, something tore loose, and words exploded.

"You wanted to tell me?" How had she gotten everything so wrong? She'd trusted him. She'd *trusted* him! But he hadn't trusted her. He hadn't told her. Perhaps he'd never meant to. Perhaps it had all been a lie. He was saying something, but she didn't want to listen, so she kept talking. "You said you loved me, but how could you love me and let me find out like this?" She flung out her hands. She'd shared *everything* with him. "Yesterday…how could you let yesterday happen without telling me?"

He looked stricken, as if he were in pain, and embarrassed, but she didn't care. He hadn't cared about her. All these weeks… What kind of man was he, to say he loved her, to *make love* to her, while pretending he didn't know her loathsome father? And now he was moving into the rapist's home. Dear God. She'd been a fool, convincing herself he'd had reasons to keep his identity secret. His lies had extended far beyond who and what he was. He was an aristocrat, with the entitlement of generations bred into him. Did they all prey upon women, use them however they wanted? She wouldn't trust him again. She struggled to breathe, to move air past the pain in her chest.

"Please, listen." With his brows furrowed, his eyes wild, Peter looked desperate. "I tried to tell you yesterday, but you wouldn't listen."

He was blaming *her*? She backed around the bed, away from Peter, keeping as far from Kenton as she could. Her eyes filled. She had to get *out*. "You're despicable," she said, hurt making the words croak.

"Don't go. Anne, listen."

She couldn't listen. Especially not with her father looking on. And with guilt hammering, because yesterday Peter had tried, again and again, to tell her something and she wouldn't let him. But he should have *made* her listen!

Peter sat up, grimacing. He dragged his legs out of bed and went still, hand pressed to his ribs. "I love you," he said, adamant almost to the point of shouting. "Anne, don't leave. We're betrothed," he said, sounding desperate. "We're *married*," he added, referencing the vows they'd exchanged.

She gasped. How dare he? She shook her head. "*No*, we are *not*." Not anymore.

He was slowly getting to his feet. She headed for the door.

Kenton spoke. "Let her go. You'll be better off. She's as flighty as her mother."

Those words stopped her, and she turned. "Stay out of this. It's none of your concern."

Kenton's head reared back. "You doubt it?" He gave a short laugh and looked toward Peter. "Be grateful. She spent her childhood pining for my love but was never brave enough to collect it—though it was always hers for the taking. Now, though she claims to love you, she's feeling sorry for herself and running away. What is that but flighty?"

Anne couldn't think. Bees buzzed in her head. It couldn't be true. It *couldn't*. But she'd heard it with her own ears.

She confronted the now standing Peter, with his desperate, wounded expression. "You told him?" Her voice came out broken, as broken as her heart. Broken trust, broken vows, broken everything.

Anne saw her words register, saw a moment of puzzlement, then Peter must have realized she meant that he'd told Kenton what she'd shared with no one but him: In spite of the evil Kenton had done, and in spite of how he'd ignored her, she'd yearned for her father's love. Peter's eyes widened and he gasped. Shock and shame filled his white face, for it was knowledge Kenton might one day use against her or her mother, who, if she ever found out, would be terribly hurt. It had been shared in confidence. Had he not realized it was something she'd never want Kenton to know? Or had he simply not cared?

Anne whirled and shot Edwin a look as she headed out the door. "I'll be back later," she said through a tight throat, and ran.

She wanted to hide. To be alone. She wanted to leave, but she couldn't. There were patients to see. So she went to Edwin's horse shed, circled behind it and sat on a tree stump. Could Peter have meant everything he said? That he loved her, that they were betrothed? Even wed? Did it matter if he meant them? Her promises had been made to a man who didn't exist. She'd told him about her mother's rape. He'd encouraged her to talk to Kenton. To have her questions answered. And he'd kissed her.

They'd been friends—closer than friends—a long while now. She might understand why he'd withheld everything in the beginning, but last week? And how could he propose without telling her about his connection to her father? She thought back. If he had told her, she'd have been too shocked and leery to accept his marriage proposal. They wouldn't have made love. He should have told her. By keeping silent, he'd betrayed her.

She covered her face with her hands, and the first sob squeezed out. She surrendered enough to let more come, each a painful wrench. How could he seek refuge at Pennyton Park, dining with Kenton, spending his leisure time with Kenton, unless... *He believed Kenton's version of what happened.* The knowledge crashed upon her like a wheelbarrow of earth upon a coffin. He'd decided Mum lied.

No. He knew her mother. How could he believe that deceitful man instead of Mum? Even if Kenton had misrepresented his account due to arrogance and denial, couldn't Peter recognize the distortion? But, then, Kenton was apparently his godfather, a close family friend. A lifelong friend. Might Peter even love him?

Her heart hurt too much to be intact. It had torn. It must have. She crossed her arms over her chest and rocked. But then a thought more hope and wish than possibility wormed its way to the forefront of her mind: What if he'd kept his secret because he loved her and couldn't bear hurting her? He'd known it would be a devastating blow. Had it been easy for her to turn him aside yesterday because he'd been afraid he'd lose her? To be fair to him, if he *had* told her, would her love have been strong enough to forgive him then? To accept him?

He'd passed her shameful confession on to Kenton, though. And now Constable Weaver, Owen Weaver, and Edwin knew, too. How much longer until her mother knew? A fresh surge of grief rose, filling her eyes and emptying her chest. Shoulders shaking, Anne squeezed her eyes closed and bent her head.

She stayed in that position for a while. No one came after her. And finally one thought prevailed, banishing all speculation: Peter wasn't the person she'd thought, and he didn't love her. Not the way she loved him. He couldn't. No heart could love both Kenton *and* her.

A short time later she heard the carriage leaving, which meant Peter was gone. Pennyton Park wasn't far, but the road was steep and rough; it would be a painful journey. Damn it! In spite of everything, she hated thinking of him in pain!

Anne moved into the horse shed and sought the solace of Snowflake, finding comfort in the affectionate mare's gentle whicker at her entrance. Scratching the mare's black, white-dappled withers eased Anne a bit. She filled her lungs again and again, willing iron into her bones, her blood, her character, and trying to subdue the storm of emotions. It seemed to take forever before she began to settle down and gain control of herself; it took longer still to turn her face into an expressionless mask, to don invisible armor, and to gather enough courage to return to the surgery.

She found Edwin and her mum drinking tea at the kitchen table. Edwin's injured ankle was propped atop a pillow on an empty chair. Mum stood and hugged Anne. Her embrace felt good. So good. Anne rested her head on Mum's shoulder and hugged her back hard.

"Edwin sent word by Michael Elmore to come," Mum said.

Anne shot Edwin a look. His quick, reassuring head shake helped her relax. She knew what it meant: Mum didn't know about Anne's old yearning. So Anne collected a cup, sat with them, and poured herself tea.

The first steaming sip tasted so good, so *normal*, she had to close her eyes and take a deep breath. But as she held the hot brew below her chin, so that the rising steam caressed her face, she realized it made no sense. On the outside everything looked, smelled, and tasted the same, but inside, nothing *felt* the same.

"I don't know how to ask," Edwin said. His chest rose with a large inhalation. "Pennyton Park has several stories and hundreds of steps. I can't manage them. Not with this pain, and on crutches. Matthews..." He stopped. "Not Matthews. Jennett. Or rather, Easterbrook," he added with an irritated-sounding sharpness. "For a time, starting tomorrow, Lord Easterbrook needs the circulation and sensation in his arm assessed. And with that rib pain, he'll have a hard time taking deep breaths. He should be watched for pneumonia. I can't do it."

"I'll go," Mum said quietly.

"What? Emma, no," Edwin said.

Anne could tell he hadn't expected Mum's offer. Neither had Anne. To think that Mum was willing to visit Pennyton to save Anne the pain of seeing Peter...

"I'll crawl up a thousand stairs before I let you step inside that place," Edwin said.

Mum reached out, and Edwin clasped her hand.

Well! Evidently some of her emotions still reacted properly, because the new unity she sensed between Mum and Edwin filled Anne with fizzy gladness. But she couldn't let Mum go to Pennyton

Park, which left only one alternative. Anne prayed she'd inherited some of the bravery she'd just seen her mum display, and dredged up every bit of single-mindedness she possessed.

"Neither Edwin's disability nor the need for Pennyton visits will last long. Not long enough to engage a temporary nurse or surgeon and get the person here," Anne said. "I'll make the Pennyton visits. All the other home visits too, of course."

Pride shone in Mum's eyes. Mutual love and pleasure warmed Anne.

"I'll take over your duties here," Mum said. "Was it really only last night that you helped me deliver the Liddle babies, Edwin?" She gave Anne a quick smile. "Unexpected twins. It was precarious for a bit, but all turned out well. That leaves only one expectant mother who is close, so working here won't be a hardship. I wish I could do more."

"I'll be fine," Anne said. She'd get in and out as fast as she could, keep herself on task while she examined Peter, and she would *not* break down.

She'd never been inside her father's summer home, and the idea was overwhelming: Possibly seeing him, in a place he felt protected and in command. Even worse, she'd see Peter, speak with him, touch him.

Mum's mouth wore a regretful twist, and she was rubbing her forehead. But there was no other option.

"It'll be fine," Anne said. Somehow, she managed to sound confident.

~

Peter looked back through the brougham window and saw his hydrangea bush, bursting with new blooms, marking the room he'd never forget. He hadn't moved the spider, who likely would now face death at the end of Mrs. Pettigrew's merciless broom.

Kenton sat beside him—quiet, thank God. Owen Weaver, who'd agreed to act as Peter's guard until his assailant had been apprehended, rode behind the lightweight carriage. Sharp arm and rib pain stabbed Peter with each jounce, but those seemed minimal compared with the rest of his misery. He barely noticed.

He was an idiot. He'd wounded the most precious person in the world. Hurt her severely, destroyed her trust—and probably love—of him. How much more horrible it all must have been for her with her father watching? Realizing Peter had told Kenton her secret had been the final devastating hurt for Anne, he realized. He remembered telling Kenton during their argument the day before. Somehow, in his anger, it had slipped out.

Peter's heart was destroyed. The empty cavity left behind had filled with excruciating pain. He didn't want to leave. He wanted to find Anne, but even if he could, he didn't think she'd listen.

Kenton gave his right forearm a pat. "It'll be all right. Anne isn't meant for you. The row with her was for the best."

Speechless, Peter stared…and saw a sympathetic if patronizing smile. Something of his shock must have shown on his face, because Kenton's brows furrowed.

"You may not feel that way now, but take my word for it. In time, you will."

"What makes you think so?"

"You need a sophisticated woman. A gentlewoman. It surprised me, I admit, your pronouncement of a betrothal. But I understand better now, why you drug up that old history the other day." He shrugged. "I'm sure she was easy to fall in love with."

"I don't care about her supposed lack of sophistication, I care about her heart. I proposed yesterday, and she accepted. I intended to tell her today about my relationship with you, but I ran out of time."

Kenton shrugged. "How could you ever have a contented marriage, disagreeing with Anne about what happened between me and her mother? Her mother has inculcated her, and your desire has blinded you. She'd never make you a suitable viscountess."

Peter stiffened, and pain bit like a knife poking between his ribs, for a moment superseding the constant ache of his other broken bones, which worsened with every jolt.

"I'll count myself fortunate if I can somehow convince her to give me another chance," he said through gritted teeth.

Kenton snorted. "You remind me of Belinda. So in love with Arthur, she refused to believe she might be happier with someone who provided a way of life similar to the one she was accustomed to."

"Belinda has a beautiful family. Arthur loves her. He's devoted to her."

"Arthur is a gentleman. The son of your father's brother. There was no valid reason to withhold my consent, although I'd hoped for a more advantageous situation for her. Anne is...well, Anne has no social standing."

Peter had assured Anne that the state of English society was changing. It was, but now that he loved her, not fast enough for him. Before Anne, Peter's opinion had been practical. Now it was personal. Kenton's viewpoint remained all too typical, and Peter was in danger of combusting.

"And yet, Anne *is* the daughter of a peer—albeit an illegitimate one who received no advantages any offspring of yours might have a right to expect."

Kenton's face flushed a dark red. He looked out the window, and a muscle at the corner of his eye twitched. "This is the steepest part of the road. I'm going to walk, give the horses some relief."

He called out to the driver, and the carriage stopped. Kenton stepped out. When the steepness eased he returned, breathing hard, to rejoin Peter. But they didn't speak for the remainder of the ride.

The brief but torturous journey to Pennyton Park finally ended. Peter wasn't sure he could stretch himself upright and walk, but he managed. He thought he might pass out before he reached the top of the stairs inside the house, but he didn't. Setting his foot on the landing, his sense of relief was immense.

Then he saw his pen-and-ink of Pennyton Park, which he'd embellished with watercolor paint. It hung at the top of the stairs, where anyone climbing the steps would see it. And Peter remembered.

Kenton had encouraged his art. Just like Anne. How could *that* man be a total monster?

CHAPTER TWENTY-EIGHT

Anne had left gauging Peter's condition for her last task of the day, and now there was nothing else to do but face him. She'd never been to Pennyton Park, one of Kenton's smaller estates with lovely hillside views, acres of pasture and even a small wood. Moss Force, a stupendous, jagged waterfall, was a short distance away.

The moment she guided Snowflake up the drive, Anne's skin became gooseflesh. She turned Snowflake over to a groom and, clutching the wide diagonal shoulder strap of her medical kit, forced her feet toward the imposing front door. The bag, similar in size to a single saddle bag, banged against her hip as she mounted the stone steps.

The ornate door opened before she rang the bell and she was ushered inside by a footman familiar to her from church services. As she entered the foyer, all the air in her lungs seemed to vanish. She ignored the chills racing down her spine and trailed the footman through the silent house, up the stairs, and into Peter's bedroom.

The footman waited near the open door while she advanced over the lush carpet to the bed. Peter appeared to be sleeping. The left sleeve of his undershirt had been cut off, providing easy access to his fractured, splinted arm. His face had a bit more color than yesterday, but new creases fanned the corners of his eyes and formed half-moon curves at the corners of his mouth.

His eyes opened, blinked. Awareness came to his gaze. She saw relief before he took a deep breath and grimaced.

"How bad is the pain?" Anne asked. She slipped her hand beneath the undershirt and gently felt the skin covering his ribs. No swelling and no popping sensation of crepitus, an indication of air in the tissue. She switched her attention to his arm, ensuring circulation above the arm splint and below, in his hand, was adequate. "Can you wiggle your fingers? Any numbness or tingling?"

He shook his head and waggled his fingers.

She could tell he hurt. Part of her wanted to lie down next to him and hold him. Comfort him and comfort herself. Instead, she pulled the covers up to his neck and straightened.

He pushed the covers to his waist and held up an imploring hand. "Please talk to me, Anne. Hear me out."

No. She wasn't talking about anything but his medical condition. His expression—he might have been a prisoner awaiting execution, begging the Lord Justice for leniency.

"When was your last dose of laudanum? How much have you had?"

His mouth tightened. His glistening eyes seemed to convey disbelief and distress. "I love you. We love each other. Please don't shut me out. Let me explain."

"I loved the man I thought you were. The man you are today… I don't know." She snapped her mouth closed. She didn't want to speak of this. Hadn't intended to.

"Please, hear me out. It all started with best intentions, and by the time I knew I needn't worry about any of you revealing who I really was, I knew the revelation would hurt you. Hurt you badly." His words rushed out, so fast they were nearly connected. "The concealment came to feel like a lie, and I hated it. Your confession that I told to Kenton? I wasn't *telling* him. When I said it, I didn't even realize what I'd done. We had a bitter argument, and it just came out."

No. She was not letting him draw her into this here. And she was not asking about the argument, even though she wanted to know. She was a nurse caring for a patient. "Who's seeing to your needs? I'll speak to him. Is it Lord Kenton's valet? Or a footman?" She stepped back.

"Don't go." Peter's face went hard and he sat up, a thin sound of pain emerging from tight lips. His head dropped, and he cradled his ribs.

"Stop it," she said. Her presence was making him worse, causing him additional pain. She had to leave, especially since her main job here was done. She whirled and hurried toward the door, stopped in front of the wide-eyed footman. "Who is caring for him?"

"Greggs, the first footman," the servant replied.

"Please find him. I'll wait downstairs."

Anne hastened out. Going down the stairs, she met Owen Weaver coming up. They both paused. Self-consciousness swamped her. Owen had been in Peter's room when all had been revealed and her world collapsed. He gave her a pointed look, and the space between his brows creased.

"Hello, Anne. Are you all right?"

"I will be." She forced a smile that felt painted on, and knew Owen must realize it wasn't heartfelt.

"I'm sorry we were there, witness to what should have been private between you and Easterbrook."

"Thank you, but you have no reason to apologize. Lord Easterbrook is to blame."

For everything.

Owen glanced up and down the stairs. "I hate that Kenton heard it all," he said with lowered voice.

Anne gave a tiny nod, acknowledging what Owen did not say. That Anne didn't want Kenton knowing her feelings, or anything else she considered her private business. Kenton's knowing she loved Peter—she especially hated that.

"You're acting in some sort of protective capacity for Lord Easterbrook?" Anne asked.

"I'm keeping an eye out, and I'll stay especially close when he leaves this house."

His jacket pocket sagged, and Anne thought it likely he carried a pistol. It gave her a bit of relief, knowing Owen was on watch, though she hated herself for caring. Peter didn't deserve her concern. All these weeks, he'd pretended. He was the only person she'd ever talked with about her mum's assault. Or about her father. She'd poured her heart out to a privileged aristocrat who believed Mum a liar and Anne naive. She'd given him honesty; he'd offered only lies.

Why, though, when all his lies were exposed, had he still professed to love her, to wanting to marry? She stiffened, slamming the door on her traitorous thoughts. The love she'd felt had been for a man who didn't exist. What did it matter if he thought he loved her? He wasn't an honorable man.

"Stay on your toes, Owen," Anne said. "Kenton and Easterbrook aren't any more trustworthy than the ruffian you're trying to catch. Easterbrook places his needs above everything else. That kind of self-importance could end up putting you in unnecessary danger."

His face scrunched up. "Well...," he said, drawing out the word, "my dealings with Easterbrook have been straightforward and he's been more than fair to me." He bent his head and rubbed the back of his neck. His face, when he lifted it, was flushed and apologetic. "I'm sorry your experience was different."

"He said you'd been working for him."

"He sent me to Cliff Gate, which is near Hawes and his ancestral home in Yorkshire. He owns a coal mine there. I snooped around a bit and identified the man I believe shot him. Unfortunately, he got wind of me and got away. Now he's here and still after Easterbrook. Monroe—that's his name—has been in hiding, and evidently he isn't aware his fellow miners are back at work."

"Did you hear about the stranger that came into the surgery a week ago?" Anne found herself saying. "Do you think he could be this man, Monroe?" Had she spoken to the very person who attacked Peter? He'd looked ordinary but had rather pointedly looked around the surgery and into the convalescent room.

Owen gave a nod. "Father is checking Braithwaite, Keswick, and the Borrowdale villages. He doesn't strike me as someone stupid enough to rent a room, though. I'm searching every outbuilding in the area a second time. He could be hiding in a barn or shed."

"I'll let you know if I notice anything unusual on my patient visits."

Owen looked concerned. "If you do see something odd, don't investigate. Leave that to me."

Anne nodded. "I'll be careful. You be careful, too."

Owen was a capable man, but the villain he sought had tried four times to commit murder. This Monroe fellow was obviously dangerous, and a man who wouldn't give up. How many times could Peter avoid misadventure before luck gave out? An icy finger traced Anne's spine and she shuddered.

"Don't worry about me. This work has brought me back to myself." Owen glanced at the pinned-up sleeve covering his stump. "I'm planning on seeking similar work in London. Easterbrook has promised to provide introductions."

"I'm glad," Anne said. The happiness his words brought were a surprising pleasure after days of emptiness and pain.

"I'll see this through first, of course." Owen Weaver's gaze swept about the open, upper area of the foyer below, skimming over portraits of people she suspected were Kenton ancestors. A couple of them had red hair like hers. "It's strange to see you in this house," he admitted to Anne.

The sound of footsteps drew their eyes downward. Lady Kenton's maid, Rosella Brown, rounded the bottom of the stairs and started up. Seeing her, Owen advanced to the next step, headed off to his probable appointment with Easterbrook.

"Take care, Anne. If you need me, I'll be here or close by."

"Good day, Owen."

He resumed his climb up the steps, and Anne headed down. Seeing her, Miss Brown stopped and waited. Anne bit back surprise. Aside from that day at the surgery, they'd never conversed, though they had often greeted each other in town and at church. When Anne drew level, the maid gave her a questioning look.

"I wasn't expecting you, Miss Albright. Did Lady Kenton request you attend her?"

What a strange question. Who could imagine Lady Kenton sending for Anne or her mother?

"No. I'm checking on Lord Easterbrook's condition. Is Lady Kenton in need of medical care?"

Miss Brown's eyelids fluttered. "Oh. No. I don't know what I'm thinking. I was just surprised to see you."

Anne hesitated, remembering her discovery of Lady Kenton's intemperance. She hated the idea the woman might have no one to turn to in a time of desperation, despite the fact that the viscountess would never be kind or grateful. "If I can ever be of help, though…to you or Lady Kenton…you can come to me," Anne said.

Miss Brown's blue eyes seemed intent as her gaze searched Anne's face. "Thank you," she said. Then her eyes fell and she proceeded up the stairs.

Anne hurried down, anxious to find Greggs and get out.

CHAPTER TWENTY-NINE

The visits got a tiny bit easier. After the first day, aside from an ignored request at the end of her visits to stay and talk, Peter had limited his conversations to answering her medical questions. She was grateful for that at least. Anne replaced her stethoscope tube in her medical kit. The past five days she'd made certain to bring the device for checking his condition. Without it, she would have to press her ear against Peter's torso in order to hear air move in and out of his lungs. She couldn't touch him so intimately and keep her shield intact; those few precious inches the listening device gave her kept the remains of her battered heart intact.

"No complications that I can detect," she said. "Is your pain under control? How often are you taking laudanum?" She picked up the laudanum bottle and eyed the contents. It was half-full.

"Three or four times a day," Peter said. "I sleep for a while after each dose."

Anne nodded. "That's fine."

She raised her kit's strap over her head, readying to leave, but Peter slowly rose from his chair, hand pressed to his ribs. "Do you have to go? Please stay and have tea. And perhaps...tell me what's in your mind and heart?"

His weary visage implored her to give him a chance. Part of her wanted that. She missed him. There wasn't a moment when she didn't feel an integral part of her was lost forever, and their estrangement was wrong. Yet another part of her condemned him as undeserving. As dishonorable.

Well, perhaps not exactly dishonorable. He'd held back his association with Kenton but not in order to take advantage of her. That day in the surgery after the attack he'd still claimed her as his wife. Over the past few days her mind had accepted that. But he had still withheld the information for far longer than she would desire from a life partner, from a man she'd need to trust implicitly for the rest of her days.

Distant but excited voices disturbed the quiet in the room. Some sort of commotion was occurring downstairs. Greggs, standing by the open bedroom door, ducked into the hall. He returned a moment later with a new air of urgency.

"I believe you could be of use downstairs, miss. If you'll come?"

Anne hurried out. Peter followed at a slower pace, but she didn't wait for him. Once upon the stairs she could see the open foyer below, and dressed in a riding habit, a distraught Belinda was at the center of a small circle of servants and her parents. Shoulders shaking, hands pressed to her eyes, she breathed like she'd run full tilt for miles.

"Tell us what's wrong!" Kenton demanded, sounding more cross than concerned.

Belinda didn't respond. Kenton gripped one of her wrists and tugged her hand away from her face, revealing her distressed expression. He pulled her other hand down, and her gaze darted around the group of watchers. Her gasping breaths didn't slow.

"Bloody hell, girl. What's happened?"

Appearing from the rear of the house, Belinda's son Henry ran to his mother and hugged her skirt and boots. Looking up he patted her arm, trying to get her attention. A housemaid carrying the baby joined them, while Lady Kenton swooped in and swept young Henry into her arms. When she straightened, she took a couple extra steps, as if correcting an off-balance sway.

"Nooooo," the boy wailed, stretching his arms toward his mother.

Gaze locked on her son, fresh tears spilled from Belinda's eyes, but she appeared too distressed to respond to him.

Anne reached the ground floor, squeezed through to her half-sister, and put a firm arm around her back. "Come sit down," she said, urging Belinda forward.

Haltingly, breathing fast and shallow as a small bird, Belinda moved. Anne propelled her toward the nearest room and located Pennyton's butler amongst those hovering nearby.

"Chamomile tea," she commanded, and with one nod from Mr. Young, a footman hurried away.

Belinda's gaze slid to Anne and latched on.

"Slow down your breathing," Anne directed as they continued across the wide foyer. "In through your nose and out through your mouth. That's it. Niiiice and slooow." Anne modeled her own breathing in the manner she wanted Belinda to follow, and kept pressing Belinda forward. Shock sometimes kept people frozen in place. At least Belinda could walk, albeit slowly.

Behind them, Lord Kenton snapped at his wife. "Can't you make him be quiet?"

"Julie," Lady Kenton said, setting Henry on his feet and holding the boy's hand toward the housemaid carrying Rebecca. "Take care of him."

The young housemaid took the boy's hand and pulled him toward the stairs.

"Nooooo," he wailed, bracing himself. But, unable to stop the forward momentum of the maid, he reluctantly followed her up the stairs, his wailing objections giving way to sobs.

"Where did Belinda go?" Kenton demanded.

"Just for a ride over the grounds," Lady Kenton responded in a placating tone. "You know she comes here and rides. Julie watches the children while she's gone."

"Well, what happened *today*?" Kenton asked. "Did she take a tumble?"

"I don't *know*," Lady Kenton snapped, sounding aggrieved.

It turned out the nearby room Anne had headed for was a sitting room. She pressed Belinda into an upholstered chair. Without Anne asking, a footman positioned another chair close. Anne sat and took Belinda's hand, which held on with a death grip.

Kenton positioned himself squarely in front of Belinda, but Anne ignored him. "You're doing better," she assured her half-sister, who'd stopped crying. "That's it. Slooow breaths in."

Belinda continued trying to match her inhalations to Anne's demonstrations. Her respiratory rate had slowed, but not enough. Peter joined them and stood beside Lady Kenton. For a brief moment, Anne's gaze connected with his. Somehow she knew the concern in his eyes wasn't only for Belinda, but herself as well.

"Enough of this," Kenton said, making an impatient gesture toward Belinda. When Belinda didn't speak, he took a step forward. "Well?"

Anne's half-sister made a sound halfway between a hiccough and a gasp. "I—I—I—" Each word was followed by a short, gasping inhalation.

"Easy," Anne cautioned. "Take your time."

"I found...Owen...Weaver." No one spoke, but they all glanced around at each other, confused. Belinda's gaze swept the faces and then stopped on Peter's. Her eyes filled with fresh tears. "He's...dead!"

A giant fist squeezed Anne's heart. No! Not Owen! She looked at Peter, who stared at Belinda with an expression of both shock and horror.

"Where?" Kenton demanded. "Where is he?"

Belinda bent her head. "The path that...goes to the...waterfall? A little ways up...Newlands Pass...from the path. In the small copse of trees...where Morse Beck branches."

Anne knew the place, the fork where one stream became two. Belinda pulled a handkerchief from her sleeve and applied it to her eyes and nose.

Kenton looked at Peter. "Your assassin did this. I'll have one man fetch Constable Weaver and your cousin, and take another with me to locate young Weaver's body. The remaining men will comb the area for the perpetrator."

Kenton strode out, and Anne found herself surprised. He was leaving without a word of comfort to his daughter? Belinda sat with bent head and closed eyes, her breaths slower but still stuttering. Anne couldn't believe that no one was offering her any sympathy.

A footman appeared with the tea cart, and Lady Kenton suddenly pressed her palm to her forehead. "I've a horrific headache. I'll take my tea in my room." Then she swept off out the door.

Anne shook her head, and she couldn't help glancing at Peter. She lifted her brows and shoulders at him: How could Belinda's parents leave when their daughter was in such a state?

Belinda released Anne's hand and raised her head. "Mother is in dire need of a laudanum dose," she explained, as if she'd heard Anne's thoughts.

Anne told the footman to pour the tea. The man didn't hesitate. Taking her direction as if she were the lady of the house, he began the ritual.

"Ma...ma...." Henry ran in, apparently having escaped the nursery. Belinda lifted him into her lap, hugged, rocked, and kissed the child. A moment later he was pushing back, struggling to get free.

"Ow. You're hurting," he cried.

Belinda released him. "Hush. Let me wipe your face." Her breathing restored to normal, she took a deep breath, released it, and mopped Henry's cheeks with her damp, crumpled handkerchief. The boy sat quietly and blew his nose when instructed.

"Look, there's cake," Belinda said to Henry. She motioned for the footman to bring her a slice.

A third chair was suddenly brought close, and Peter sat with a weary-sounding sigh. They soon had steaming cups in front of them, and Henry was happily consuming his sweet and Anne was wondering at how strange it was that everyone was acting like business as usual. Well, except for the tea. Chamomile would be good for Belinda, but Anne wished hers was the usual, bracing variety.

"What a tragedy," Peter said, sorrow lacing his words. "He was a good man." He raked his hand through his hair. "I wish I was in a state to go and see what happened." He looked at Anne. "He was your friend."

Anne nodded. "I can't remember when he wasn't. The last few times I saw him, he seemed to be adjusting to the loss of his arm. I was so glad of that. I think the work you gave him helped."

Peter's mouth went tight. "I wish I'd never hired him. He'd be alive today."

"We've all done things we regret," Belinda said. "It'll do no good to chastise yourself."

As Anne's half-sister smoothed the dark hair on the crown of her child's head, Anne's mind jumped to the way Peter had asked over and over for an opportunity to explain his mistakes with her. He'd said he was desperate, that he wanted to heal their rift, that he wasn't giving up. She'd been so angry but…she really did want him to explain. If he died tomorrow, she knew, she'd be very sorry she never gave him the chance.

Julie the nursemaid returned, and this time Henry, replete with cake and tea, accompanied her willingly. A somber silence fell, broken only by the occasional clink of china. Peter and Belinda seemed lost in reflection. Anne's thoughts spun like a child's top. Finally she bent her head, prayed for the soul of Owen and his family, and let herself relax.

Eventually they heard voices, and Rector Jennett strode into the room. He went straight to his wife.

"Arthur!" Belinda stood, and they embraced.

Anne recalled the day she'd seen Belinda and Richard Thorpe together in Danvers Retail and thought them flirtatious. At the time it had made her wonder if the Jennett marriage was all it should be. Today Belinda held her husband and pressed against him, appearing grateful for his presence and as in love with him as any wife could be. It relieved Anne, to conclude the exchange she'd witnessed must have been a simple teasing between old friends. She was glad she hadn't related the incident to Peter or anyone else, and she rose and moved to the other side of the room to give the couple some semblance of privacy.

Peter joined her.

"Are you all right?" Mr. Jennett was asking his wife. Belinda didn't reply, and he repeated his question, a bit louder and with more emphasis.

"Yes," Belinda said. She didn't step back but clung to her husband. "Oh, Arthur. It was so horrible." Face pressed to her husband's chest, she began to cry again. Standing strong and steady, Mr. Jennett rocked his wife and murmured in her ear. After a short while, Belinda quieted.

"Your father sent a groom to fetch me," Mr. Jennett said, "and I nearly lost my mind when I understood what had occurred. I rode with Constable Weaver and we met your father and his party on the way. We prayed over Owen's body, then I came on here while Weaver stayed behind."

Belinda released her husband but continued to stand close to him.

"It seemed to take forever to get here," Jennett said. "All I could think of was you, in those trees with a killer. What if you'd happened upon him in the act?" He drew Belinda into another embrace. "He might have killed you," he said in an agonized whisper.

Anne looked at Peter, who studied the carpet. Her stomach gave a sharp squeeze as she was reminded that he was the man the killer intended to dispatch. No matter her anger at his mistakes, she couldn't imagine a world without him in it.

"Weaver will need to ask you some questions, dearest," Mr. Jennett said as he and Belinda stepped apart. "Probably not many for now. It'll be even harder on him than you."

Belinda nodded. The rector pulled a handkerchief from his coat and gently dried her tears. She gave a tiny smile.

"Shall I ask your mother to take Henry for the night? We can have a cold supper and go to bed after you nurse Rebecca and put her down."

"No. I want them both with us. It'll be a comfort, the children being their normal selves."

Anne felt uneasy. The pair seemed to have forgotten they weren't alone. She thought she and Peter should leave, but then Mr. Jennett looked their way.

"Let's sit down," he said, with a wave including Peter and Anne.

Belinda clutched her husband's arm. "Wait." She turned her back to Anne and looked up at her husband. "Do I seem...myself?" she asked in a low voice. "I feel...unhinged."

Oh, dear. Anne could still hear her, and this sounded like a conversation one held in private. She glanced at Peter, who wore an enigmatic expression. He smiled, though, and she knew it was because he approved of the very obvious love his cousin and her half-sister shared.

Mr. Jennett frowned and studied his wife's face. "You don't have any color in your cheeks." His forehead smoothed. "Once we're home, a glass of sherry wouldn't be amiss."

Belinda licked her lips. "I mean...do you still love me?"

Anne frowned. Her half-sister's tone begged for reassurance, as if finding Owen's body had changed her in some elemental way. It must have been awful, of course. Belinda made a good accounting of herself when she helped after the natural deaths of community members, but murder was something else entirely.

Mr. Jennett hugged his wife and gave a gentle laugh. "Of course I love you. This has been even more of a shock than I realized if you could ask that." He looked at Anne and Peter and smiled.

Outside, several voices could be heard shouting for all to keep a sharp eye and about Lord Kenton wanting the grounds searched. Anne had a sudden thought: After the way Belinda's parents had acted today, it was no mystery why she needed to hear her husband loved her.

CHAPTER THIRTY

The next day Peter couldn't turn his mind to his architecture books or even to the book of William Wordsworth's poetry he'd borrowed from the manor library and was enjoying immensely. Instead he brooded and scribbled drawings that did nothing to relieve his tension. His forced inactivity and isolation had never sat so heavy as today.

Yesterday, after talking with Belinda, Constable Weaver had left to attend to his wife, Owen's body, and the enlistment of additional men to search for the killer. When Kenton returned from the site of the crime, he'd told Peter what little he knew and that they were to expect Weaver back today. When the constable finally strode through Peter's bedroom door with Kenton following, the wave of relief was instantaneous. Then grief tempered his sense of deliverance.

Kenton and Weaver took chairs opposite Peter's chaise.

"May I offer my deepest sympathy, Constable," Peter said. "Owen was a son to be proud of. That he was killed while in my service is something I'll always regret. Did he have a wife or children? I'd be honored to provide a monthly pension."

"Thank you." The creases, the very skin of Weaver's face, seemed to have sagged since the last time Peter saw him. But then the constable shook his head and added, "He was unmarried. And if you harbor any guilt, my lord, discharge it now. Owen came back to himself after you hired him. When he returned from Cliff Gate, he'd decided investigative work suited him. He'd regained his dignity and pride. I'll always be grateful you saw more than an incapacitated, melancholy, one-armed veteran."

Peter sighed. While he understood and appreciated Weaver's sentiments, they didn't entirely mitigate his sense of blame. "I came to Pennyton because I wanted to keep Miss Albright and Carter out of harm's way, and I believed I'd be protected here. Now Owen is dead, and I realize I underestimated my enemy. I think it's best I go to Treewick Hall, where only my own people will be in danger. I *will* assemble a team to find and capture Monroe, though." He hoped the look he leveled at Weaver conveyed his determination. "I'm committed to finding him. He's a murderer now, and when he's caught, he'll hang. This heinous crime—Owen's murder—will not be forgotten."

The tightness of Weaver's mouth eased a bit. He nodded.

Kenton scraped his fingers through his hair. "You stand a better chance of catching him here, Peter. We *know* he's around, and he's likely desperate. I have a lot of staff—year-round groundskeepers and those I employ for the horse breeding—plus additional grooms and house servants while I'm in residence. I've got all the outdoors help armed and posted, encircling the house. Inside, two men will be on watch around the clock: one just outside your room and another downstairs. Weaver has alerted the community. Everyone's got their eyes open.

"And...I've an idea." He glanced at Weaver. "We'll set a trap." He leaned forward. "And *get* him."

A trap? Peter nodded, bristling with anger. "I'll be the bait? That's a good idea." If only he were fit enough to turn from quarry to hunter. He wanted the opportunity to get in a few licks.

Weaver rubbed the back of his neck. "I've some reservations, but we could turn something as simple as a daily constitutional to our advantage. Stay close to the mansion, where there're outbuildings and natural cover for the men, and position them along the route. We'll be close, and you'll be armed."

"I'll walk slow, which I need do anyway, and dangle the bait." Peter glanced out the window. He couldn't wait to get on with it.

"Anne would make an excellent addition," Kenton said. "If she were with you, the outlaw would have little reason to be suspicious."

The idea was like a slap; outrage exploded in Peter's head. "She'd be in danger!"

"Not much," Kenton replied.

Putting any woman in danger was wrong, but Anne? Unthinkable.

"How can you even consider putting your own daughter in the killer's path?"

He hadn't realized he'd spoken aloud until Kenton's head jerked and his eyes narrowed. The viscount went still, and nothing but his lips moved. "If she cared about you, she'd want to do it."

Anne's desire to help wasn't a consideration. What struck Peter most was that Kenton had no tender feelings for Anne. None. So smart and brave, kind and beautiful. So deserving of love, and so very lovable. Granted, the pair had enjoyed little interaction since her birth; the viscount had done no more than impregnate Anne's mother, but didn't he feel *some* pride at all she'd accomplished? Did he even regard her as his daughter? This was yet another act of his godfather that made him think he'd misjudged the man all along.

"I'll walk alone," Peter declared. "That will be equally disarming. Perhaps a stroll after dinner before I turn in. I'm sure the killer will feel safer in the shadows."

Weaver stood. "I think this has a good chance of catching him."

"I know just where to place watchers. Let's go to the library and I'll lay out the plan for you. All you need do is make certain your men don't botch the job," Kenton commanded, and the pair headed out toward the hall, Constable Weaver looking aggrieved.

Peter watched his godfather's back recede. Once he'd believed in Kenton's innocence, or at least mitigating circumstances, but the more he watched the man's behavior, the more doubt seeped in and coalesced in his belly. Kenton was arrogant, so certain he knew the right of everything, and he had not a shred of sympathy for anyone. Why hadn't Peter seen that before? And why hadn't he asked Arthur's view? His cousin knew his godfather very well, was an astute judge of character, and would have every reason to believe in the innocence of his wife's father—if it was possible, which Peter doubted more and more. Had Arthur ever come to a verdict on Kenton's innocence?

Peter was going to find out.

~

His cousin arrived for a visit late the following morning, an Arthur with new facial lines and plodding tread.

"You look as if you need coffee," Peter said. "Did you sleep?" He called out for Greggs, the footman, now armed and always within earshot, who appeared in the doorway. Peter requested sandwiches and coffee.

Arthur dropped heavily into one of the comfortable chairs near Peter's chaise and rubbed his temples like they ached. His hands moved to cup the top of his head, and Peter got a good look at his cousin's eyes, which were haunted. "Belinda's been acting strange."

Peter said nothing, just waited for Arthur to continue.

"I understand finding young Weaver's body shocked and disturbed her, but even so her reaction seems extreme." Arthur's hands dropped to his sides. "Both nights she watched the children sleep, and didn't sleep herself. She refused to come to bed. This morning she almost seems to be sleepwalking. She withdraws into her thoughts and doesn't hear the children. She's scaring me. Nothing I do seems to help." Peter's cousin's eyes and lips squeezed into tight slashes. "She won't *talk* to me."

Peter didn't know what to say. "Was Weaver a good friend of hers?"

"She knew him, of course, but he wasn't a special friend." Arthur opened his hands as if in supplication. "I don't understand it."

"Being alone and finding someone who met his end through violence, knowing the perpetrator could be hiding and watching...it would unsettle any lady," Peter suggested. Except Anne. He couldn't imagine her being cowed by such a situation. She was fearless—and unforgiving.

Arthur sighed. His shoulders sagged, and he seemed to shrink. His eyes begged, but what did his cousin need? Understanding? Reassurance? Advice? Arthur wanted answers, but Peter had none.

"Last week she apologized for being erratic and melancholic. Said she'd tried to control or hide her moods and couldn't." Arthur hesitated. His voice dropped to a low whisper. "And now *this*. Should Carter attend her, do you suppose?" One hand opened and closed nervously. "I'm so afraid...her mind may have snapped."

The statement brought Peter up short. He rose—slowly, because of rib pain—and moved toward his cousin, who stood when Peter drew close. Peter gripped his shoulder. Arthur's eyes glistened.

"Are you worried she might endanger the children?" If Belinda was altered to such a degree that she posed a risk to her family, the situation was dire. And tragic. There wouldn't be much, if anything, any physician could do.

"Not because of any design to do so. But perhaps, because of inattention...." Arthur's voice trailed off. "Today I was afraid to leave her but felt compelled to seek your guidance."

The coffee and sandwiches arrived, and both men went quiet. Arthur retook his seat, sinking into its cushions with a defeated-sounding moan, and Peter returned to the chaise. Once served, Peter asked Greggs to close the door behind him.

"Eat something and get some coffee in you," he commanded his cousin. "You need it."

Arthur appeared to agree, because for a few minutes he attended to the food and drink. How strange, that his cousin had come for his advice when Peter very much wanted Arthur's in return.

"Might you appeal to her mother?" he asked. "Perhaps the children could stay here for a time, or a housemaid could be sent to the rectory to mind the children." And if Belinda's needs were beyond what a rest would provide, Peter didn't know what to suggest. The care and supervision of an asylum were a disagreeable matter altogether, and if necessary, the future of Arthur's marriage and family were uncertain at best.

"Belinda's funny about leaving the children here. She's worked hard to be independent and as capable as she thinks a rector's wife should be...," Arthur said, shaking his head as if bewildered. "After four years of marriage, she still fears disappointing me. Still needs my praise and reassurance."

"Really?" That came as a surprise. Peter had always thought Belinda very sure of herself.

"When we met, I was struck by how much love she had to give. And how starved for love she seemed."

"Why is that, do you think?" Peter asked.

A long moment passed before Arthur replied. "I know how much you admire Kenton, but he and Belinda's mother were neither loving nor attentive parents. Not to any of their brood. How did they act yesterday, when Belinda arrived?"

"Honestly? Inconvenienced and annoyed." As much as Peter hated to admit it, for it underlined all his current misgivings.

"I know plenty of titled parents leave the childrearing to the nurse, and later, the tutor or governess. That may be fine for some children, but I think it was detrimental to Belinda. She's sensitive. Her self-worth has improved since our marriage, but she used to have quite a low opinion of herself. While to others she seems confident, she is in fact very unsure of herself." The corners of Arthur's lips curved. "She's probably the most tenderhearted person I've ever known. She lives for me and the children. She's dedicated herself to this community too, trying to prove herself, yet she's still perceived as arrogant. She's not. I think she distances herself because she's afraid of being hurt." Peter's cousin filled his chest with air, held it a moment, and let it out. "Children need love, and I fear Belinda didn't receive any. Deep inside, she feels unworthy of it."

"I'm sorry," Peter said, meaning it. "She believes you love her, I hope?"

Arthur nodded. "She says, before our marriage she never realized the bond between husband and wife could be so deep and strong, but

I had a struggle convincing her I love her. Even now it's all too easy for doubts to creep in. I haven't asked for, nor do I want perfection, but she wears herself to a frazzle trying to be the consummate rector's wife and mother."

"To be affected so profoundly...do you think her parents did something worse than ignore her?"

Arthur thought about that longer than Peter would have liked.

"According to Belinda, nothing she did pleased her father. She had a strict governess who used discipline too harsh for a young girl. It was downright cruel. I blame Kenton for letting it go on. He approved of using a stern hand. He condoned—even encouraged—the discipline. She expected nothing but condemnation from him."

"He spent so much time writing to me," Peter said, truly confused. "His letters were full of encouragement and praise. I don't understand."

"Nor do I, but I think his sons enjoyed more privilege than his daughters. Especially Robert, the heir. And you were already a viscount when your correspondence began."

Peter shivered. It filled him with cold, thinking Kenton might show a different side to his daughters and wife, whose lives were dependent on his largesse. They'd come to this topic in a different way than Peter had imagined, but he intended taking advantage of the opportunity. "Did you ever wonder if Emma Albright's claim is true?"

Arthur's eyes closed, and he dragged his hand over his lower face. When his gaze returned to Peter, it was tortured.

"I've wondered, and I don't know. I'm accountable for every soul in this parish, and that includes Kenton and Mrs. Albright. If her charge is true, there are actions I should take. I fear God is disappointed in me. I've prayed for guidance, for Him to show me the truth, but I'm no closer now than I was when I arrived in Buttermere."

Arthur's words chilled Peter to his core. This was hardly close to an exoneration.

"What does Belinda say?" he asked.

"She says Emma is lying. Belinda even claims she's uncertain Kenton fathered Anne."

"But their eyes. And he admitted to being Anne's father. How can Belinda doubt it?"

Arthur shook his head and shrugged. "I suppose because she doesn't want to accept it."

"When Father died," Peter said, a myriad of emotions rising like bile from a putrid stomach, "Kenton became the one whose counsel I sought as I took on the duties of the title. Have I been denying what I didn't want to believe, just as Belinda has? Everything I've learned tells me Kenton is generous with his money but stingy with his heart. His largesse seems to stem not from a desire to help, but from a need to be admired and for others to feel obligated to him. I wonder if Father realized the kind of person his friend was. He must have had these same attributes as a young man, when their friendship was established...?"

"I like to think Uncle John wouldn't have named Kenton your godfather if he doubted his integrity. But Kenton is different with some people than others. He doesn't always show his most offensive traits."

A sweaty fist squeezed Peter's heart and lungs. "I didn't see them until just recently." "Well, you're running straight and true now, and the blinkers are off," Arthur said. He sounded sad.

"I suppose I should be pleased you likened me to a race horse rather than a donkey."

Peter's cousin shot him a glance that clearly questioned whether he was unbalanced, but then he half smiled. "I'd never liken you to a donkey. There wasn't an eyelash of donkey in Aunt Julia, and I'm positive the Jennett lineage is donkey free. I am your cousin, after all."

Peter could always depend on Arthur to take his side. But... "I'm very much afraid I have been a donkey lately."

Arthur tugged his ear. "Kenton's done enormous good. It's all too easy to see his accomplishments and not what's behind them. It's never comfortable or enjoyable seeing the dark side of someone who matters to you." He paused. "In the case of my father-in-law, *I'm* still not exactly sure what's in the man's heart. At least you have the excuse of having had more of a long-distance acquaintance and seldom being in his presence." Arthur set his cup and saucer down and stood. "I should go."

Peter locked his hand with his cousin's for a long, unifying moment, and then he spoke the truest words he'd said in a long time. "I'm glad you came. Whatever happens, don't ever think you've disappointed God. You never could."

CHAPTER THIRTY-ONE

A jumble of emotions warred within Anne's chest as she followed the footman to Peter's bedroom. After almost two weeks, Edwin's ankle pain and swelling were mostly gone; he planned to resume home visits tomorrow. Even if he hadn't been fit, Peter's injuries no longer required close observation; he was apparently taking evening walks around the grounds. So, this could be the last time she ever saw him, and the realization made Anne feel like a goose about to slide into an oven, stuffed to bursting with regret and sorrow and loss.

Each visit had been exhausting and painful, but by mustering every bit of will she possessed, she'd managed to conceal how they affected her. Today's visit would be the worst of the lot, and perhaps her last opportunity to let him explain his mistakes.

She expected her heart's usual painful pinch when she saw him sitting in a chair at the window, but the pinch strengthened into something more like a fatal stab. She froze and her face must have alerted him, because he stood.

"Today's my final day here. You no longer need daily checks, besides which, Edwin is resuming his normal activities."

Peter seemed suddenly determined. He crossed the room and waved the waiting footman back into the hall. "We'll have tea, Greggs," he said, and shut the door.

The click of the latch revived Anne. What did he think he was doing? "Open that door."

"No. We need to talk."

A surge of hope went through her, but she ruthlessly crushed it. "Why am I surprised you have no care for my reputation?"

He scowled. "This is more important than silly servants' gossip."

"An aristocrat would think his need more important than anything else, but I assure you it is *not*," Anne snapped. She opened the door, pulling so hard it flew from her hand and hit the wall with a bang. Then she folded her arms.

She'd expected the action to make him furious, but the corners of his mouth edged up and his eyes gleamed. Heat suffused her. She wanted to kick him. Among other things.

The look of pleasure dropped from his face, and intensity appeared. "Nothing is more important than you hearing what I have to say. The first day you came to Pennyton, you made it clear you didn't want to talk. So I haven't pressed. We both had things to think through, and I wanted you to come to me when you were ready. I've appreciated and hated the discomfort I know you feel while being in Pennyton attending me."

Anne had been both grateful for and annoyed by his patience, but she appreciated him acknowledging the difficulty of coming here. And yes, she was finally ready to listen. They had wasted more than enough time. She gave a nod.

Peter's entire body seemed to slacken, and the tension in his face eased. He waved toward the sitting area at the other side of the room. "Would you care to sit?"

Knowing he would sit beside her, she chose the divan. It was a bold move, and her heartbeat quickened. She wanted to be close, to be able to look into his eyes when he said whatever it was that needed saying. It might be the last words they ever spoke.

Or perhaps not.

Peter sat and took a moment, looking down and seeming to gather his thoughts. Finally he sighed and looked up, saying, "I've been an arrogant arse. When you told me about Kenton, it took a long while before I sincerely considered the possibility your accusations could be true. I struggled."

Anne grew warm and wished she'd left the door closed. His voice was barely above a whisper, and she had to lean in to hear him, which positioned her too close, bringing into sharp focus the dark gray rings that circled the blue of his eyes and filling her nose with the light, clean scent of his soap. And he'd begun by saying all the right things.

He cupped her left upper arm and continued. "I'm sorry. To the bottom of my soul, I am sorry." He gave her arm a gentle squeeze. "I have serious doubts about my godfather, and I'm going to get to the truth."

A surge of pleasure sent tingles cascading down Anne's spine. Peter's hand was warm, his hold light. She wanted his arms wrapped around her; she yearned to be in his embrace. A wild bud of hope burst within her chest, but she squashed it. He was only "going to get to the truth." That didn't change anything.

"I'm glad of that," she said. "But it doesn't change what happened. Your secrets. So many secrets." Wouldn't she be a fool to trust him again?

A red wash stained his cheeks. "A different name and standing in society don't change who I am inside," he said. Releasing her, he pressed his palm to his chest. His voice went deep and fierce. "I'm the same man. The man who loves you and wants you for his wife. The man who won't take no for an answer."

Anne's ebbing anger surged and crashed like surf in a storm. "Won't take no? So I have no choice in the matter?" Was his skepticism of Kenton mere pretense? A way to gain her favor? Even if Peter was sincere, he was showing the same aristocratic arrogance that she loathed in her father.

Peter's eyes narrowed, and his mouth went tight as if he were in pain. He straightened, which increased the distance between them. "I hoped you'd sort this out by now. If I thought it would help, I'd beg. I love you. I don't know how to convince you."

"*I* should sort it out? I'm in the wrong, am I, by not seeing reason?" Anne clutched her head. It felt in danger of bursting. She pressed the heels of her hands into her eyes. Breathed. Slow and precise, she added, "You've apologized for being an arse but haven't stopped being one."

Silence. She let her hands drop and opened her eyes. His temple pulsed and the space between his brows creased. They stared at each other, and her anger drained away as she saw the hurt pouring through him. She'd tried not to, but she still loved him. She loved deeply...but that didn't mean they belonged together.

"I'm glad you want the truth about Kenton," she said.

Peter gave a nod, put his hand in his pocket and sighed. "I have been a donkey. Again. I do want the truth about Kenton. And I do want you—but I don't say that I deserve you. I'll be patient for as long as it takes for us to work this through, for it will always be your decision if we wed. And if we don't work it through...well, I'll become the most patient man on earth. I will only marry the brilliant young woman who nursed me back to health and taught me to be me. No other woman will do."

Anne stifled a laugh and glanced at his opposite hand, where his fingers protruded from the edge of his sling. Their color and size appeared normal. She'd half known she hadn't needed to come today, except she'd had to see him one more time. All while hoping for this. Wasn't this what she was hoping for?

"If I have someone drive me into town, will you see me?" Peter asked. "Join me for tea, perhaps, or a meal?"

Her heart rocked like a lifeboat on a rocky sea. Was it truly possible they could have a future together? This wasn't the same man she'd rejected. He wanted to know the truth about Kenton, and he'd just reaffirmed that he loved her and wanted them to marry. But she'd also had more time to think. If by some miracle he overcame her objections, it would mean leaving Buttermere and being a viscountess, which she had no idea how to go about. Was that part of what kept her from saying yes?

"You can't possibly believe I was taking advantage of you," Peter said in a cautious tone. "But how can I prove my feelings are sincere?"

When she'd learned who he was, there'd been a moment when she wondered if he'd lied in order to take advantage of her. Except, no matter what her reasoning suggested, her heart refuted her mind. He'd omitted—lied—about so much, but in spite of those lies, she trusted that he felt the same for her as she felt for him. And he kept speaking of marriage. What point was there in that if he didn't mean it?

In the beginning, those early hours when he'd clung to life, they'd been patient and nurse. As his condition improved, he'd become a man who enjoyed listening while she read Dickens aloud, or one who schemed to improve the life of Michael Elmore, or who faced her across a backgammon board, or who shared simple companionship and misery at the loss of her patients. He'd become a fine artist with a handsome face and a multitude of sweet words. It had been more than two months, and she'd seen him every day. He was *that* man, and it didn't matter if he was a commoner or a viscount.

He waited for her answer.

"No need," she said. "I believe you."

His lips curved and his eyes grew warm.

The footman—Greggs—strode in with a tray laden with tea and other accoutrements, which reminded Anne of her own duty. She reached for her medical bag, which she'd placed at her feet. After asking Greggs to pour, she checked Peter's arm, his ribs, and his breathing. And she thought about what would come next.

"You're healing well. Faster than I expected. Your lungs expand nicely and sound clear, thanks in part to the deep breathing regimen you practiced in spite of your rib pain."

"My daily constitutional has contributed, I think."

"Yes, I've heard you've been walking the grounds. Navigating the stairs hasn't been a problem?" That surprised her, what with injured ribs, but he was right that the activity would have promoted lung health and increased his strength and stamina.

"I've been doing my part trying to catch Owen's murderer. We set a trap for the rat, but he hasn't taken the cheese. He's likely left the area, I suppose. Every effort to find him has failed."

Anne was glad that they were trying to catch Monroe, but a sudden realization made her angry. "Don't tell me *you* were the cheese."

The block-head smiled, though his eyes remained serious. "Who better?

"But, you aren't fit to defend yourself."

"I had plenty of men watching, ready to come to my aid: Richard Thorpe and his father, the grooms and groundskeepers, and Greggs and other footmen handy with a firearm."

That information soothed her somewhat. "Kenton hires trustworthy people, I'm told. He demands nothing but the best, which he feels is his due."

Peter pressed his lips together, a narrow rift surrounded by what was now a short, neatly trimmed beard and mustache. She expected him to object, but he surprised her and said, "I saw that for myself recently. It made me take a hard look at a lot of things."

He didn't add more, and they fell silent.

She intended to take no more than a few sips of tea, but in seeking a neutral topic for a few minutes' discussion she asked what he was reading and was delighted to discover they were both enjoying her favorite poet, William Wordsworth.

"He lived in Grasmere, you know," she said. "Less than fifteen miles away. He's buried there at St. Oswald's."

"Did you ever meet him?" Peter asked.

"When I was fourteen. I was flustered, and he was kind. He gifted me with a volume of his *Guide to the Lakes* and inscribed it. I cherish it."

"I'd certainly prize such an item," Peter said.

Anne finished her tea, having stayed much longer than intended. But she had other rounds to make, other work to do.

As she prepared to leave, Peter stood. “I’m determined to erase your doubts, Anne. I don’t care how long it takes. I’m not giving up.” He paused, his mouth curving slightly. “Wordsworth said, ‘What we need is not the will to believe, but the wish to find out.’ I have that wish, and I’m going to learn the truth.”

Anne did not comment, but she left the room with a new lightness inside her.

CHAPTER THIRTY-TWO

The lightness lasted until she reached the landing, where she found Rosella Brown pacing, a frown of worry and tension on her face. Anne started to speak, but she stopped when Rosella's eyes widened with a look of alarm. The maid held her finger to her lips in a silent warning to be quiet, Anne gave a terse nod, and Rosella waved for her to follow down the north hall.

Anne didn't move. Guest rooms stretched behind her down the south hall, so, unless she was mistaken, and she knew she was not, the family bedrooms were situated off the north hallway.

Rosella had started to walk, but now she retraced her steps. She waited, and her eyes were pleading. Anne read the maid's lips as she silently begged, *Please*.

Anne had no business in the family wing. She didn't *want* to go there. Except, Rosella's distress wouldn't let her refuse.

The maid grasped Anne's hand, pulled, and Anne let herself be swept along in the maid's wake. They didn't slow until they approached an open door at the end of the hall. Rosella stopped short of that door and pulled Anne next to the wall.

Kenton's voice, resonating with disgust, carried down the hall.

"I'm sick to death of you, you wretched bitch."

Rosella's worried blue eyes fixed on Anne. Was the viscount speaking to the viscountess? Why else would the lady's maid have brought her, except out of concern for her mistress?

His next words confirmed it.

"You're no better than a bloody opium eater. Barely able to walk and talk. I should find you a friendly opium den. You could disappear forever."

Cold swept over Anne's shoulders and down her arms. Should she go after Peter? Wouldn't hearing Kenton speak to his wife this way help persuade him that his godfather was a different man than he imagined?

"Where is that bloody maid? Brown!" Kenton bellowed.

Rosella gave Anne a huge-eyed look of dismay and hurried into the room.

"Your lordship—"

"She's stupefied," the viscount accused. "I told you to search her clothing, her bags, her trunk. You were to search *everywhere*. You assured me she didn't have any laudanum."

Anne looked in the direction of Peter's room, but the bristling anger in Kenton's voice held her feet in place. He sounded on the verge of losing control. What if the women needed her help?

"Last month, while you were gone, Lady Kenton had a megrim. She insisted on obtaining laudanum from Mr. Carter, but I've kept the bottle with me. I suspect she somehow acquired another bottle, but she denies it."

"You suspected? You're either the most naive or the stupidest woman I've ever employed. Look at her! It's obvious she has a bottle of her own, now, isn't it? You're discharged."

"Noooo. You can't turn her out," Lady Kenton objected, words slow, slurred, and emphatic. "I need her."

"Drink more of your tonic," Kenton taunted. "You won't miss her."

"I *need* my tonic, you bastard. It helps me forget I'm married to *you*."

"My lord," Rosella said in a rush, "she doesn't mean it. She's not herself."

"*You* get out," Kenton ordered. "Go pack your bag. You're leaving tonight." A moment of silence, then he yelled, "*Go*."

Rosella fled into the hallway and straight to Anne.

"Fetch Lord Easterbrook," Anne whispered urgently. Rosella hurried away, and a few feet from the landing broke into a run.

"Where's that bottle?"

The menacing tone of Kenton's voice made Anne shudder. She heard him moving about in the room, the thud of something hitting the floor, and the slam of a chest.

"Stop it!" Lady Kenton shrilled. "No! Stop!"

In quick succession Anne heard muffled exclamations from Kenton, the rip of tearing fabric, the sharp sound of a slap. Then the unmistakable sounds of china breaking and a body hitting the floor.

Anne jolted into action before she thought. One moment she stood in the hall, the next she stood in the viscountess's sitting room. Near a dark green divan, Lady Kenton struggled up to her elbow from the floor. Lord Kenton stood near her, watching. A tea cart sat before the window. A small, overturned table surrounded by scattered blue-and-white-patterned china lay next to the viscountess. Anne had a momentary impression of dark paisley upholstered chairs, gleaming tables, and the scent of fresh roses.

Anne hurried to the viscountess. "Are you all right?"

Lady Kenton didn't answer, just pushed up to her knees and tried to rise. Anne helped her, and the viscountess immediately sank onto the divan and buried her face in her hands.

"Bloody hell!" Kenton swore.

Standing mere feet away, the man seemed to expand, growing taller and broader. With flushed face and clenched fists, he looked ready to explode. His torn pocket dangled.

"You." He pointed his finger at Anne. "Get out," he snapped, all the more fearsome for his biting control. Temple pulsing, he took a step forward, which brought him far too close. Anne's heart hammered. The urge to collapse onto the divan and cower beside the viscountess was strong, but instead she locked her knees.

"You need to leave so I can tend to Lady Kenton," Anne said. "She's beside herself."

Kenton's glaring eyes spat fire. His lips drew back from clenched teeth. "If you don't go, you'll be very sorry you didn't."

Was he threatening physical harm, or retribution? The only witness was the recently struck, distraught Lady Kenton, whose face remained hidden behind her hands.

Kenton's sizable left hand gripped Anne's arm. Shocked, she stared in disbelief at the gold signet ring glinting on his pinky. Fear twisted her stomach and turned her cold as he pulled. He was going to toss her out! Anne resisted, leaning away. His grip tightened, tugged and lifted, and forced her onto her toes.

"What's going on?"

Peter. Thank God. Back straight, shoulders broad, he strode in without the slightest sign of disablement, and Kenton released Anne and took a step back. Kenton waved a hand dismissively, but his mouth remained ugly-tight and his eyes glittered. Anne sensed that behind those probing eyes her father's mind churned like a bonfire in a whirlwind.

"Nothing," he said. "Nothing you need attend to."

Peter frowned. Lady Kenton raised her head. One side of her face was crimson. Peter's gaze moved to Anne and lingered an extra moment. Anne saw Rosella stood just outside the doorway, in the shadowy hall, hands clasped at her waist, shifting from one foot to the other.

"This doesn't look like nothing," Peter said.

The two men shifted and came face-to-face. Kenton's head tipped to the side and he said, "I'm sure you understand." He smiled benignly, a lauded professor explaining an important principle to a student. "I don't tolerate interlopers in my personal business... Not a nurse or a maid." A moment passed. "Not even you."

The two men seemed to take each other's measure, then Kenton shrugged. "A man has the right to take his wife to task. Especially in his own house."

"I heard you threaten Anne. You had hold of her."

Kenton's brows rose. "She deserves more than threats, sneaking about my house, insinuating herself into private affairs. All without invitation or justification."

Rosella made a small sound and moved into the room. They all turned to look, and Kenton frowned as the maid said, "I was afraid, so I fetched Miss Albright." Her voice begged for understanding. There was no defiance, nothing but a sad, knowing finality in her speech. Her shoulders squared. "I had to."

Kenton gave a deep chuckle and leveled a mere second's challenging gaze on Peter. "I hope you don't question my right to discharge unsatisfactory help?" A moment later he settled an intimidating glower on Rosella. "Don't bother appealing to Mrs. Fairchild for references or this month's wages. You didn't finish the month. There's nothing owed you."

The knuckles of Rosella's clasped hands turned white. "I knew it was naught but a matter of time before I was either gone from your service or my lady was gone to her grave, my lord."

The droopy viscountess came to life. She stood, weaved, and grabbed her husband's arm. "Nooo. You're not discharging Brown. I won't let you."

Kenton jerked his arm away and gave his wife a blistering look when she clutched the back of the divan. "I'll find someone suitable when we return to London. Until then, you can make do."

"Good-bye, my lady." Rosella turned away.

With a strangled cry, Lady Kenton unsteadily followed her maid, hands working at the clasp of her necklace. "Wait. Take this." She extended the pendant and chain she'd removed. When Rosella didn't take them, Lady Kenton grabbed the maid's hand, placed the pendant and chain in her palm, and curled Rosella's fingers over them. When Kenton started across the room, Lady Kenton gave Rosella a push.

"It's yours," she said. "Now go."

The maid threw Peter a pleading look and dashed away. Kenton grabbed his wife's arm and jerked her from the doorway. Pulled off balance she stumbled, and Kenton pulled her up with a second jerk. She cried out and went stiff.

"Bloody hell, James," Peter said. He strode to Kenton and seized his wrist. "You're hurting her."

For a moment the two men stared at one another. Kenton didn't release his viscountess, but tension left his arm, and Lady Kenton's posture slackened into something more natural appearing. Peter's hand fell.

"Have you lost your mind?" Kenton demanded of his wife. "That pendant cost more than Brown makes in a year."

Lady Kenton pulled free and stepped away. She grabbed the back of a chair. "Take it out of my pin money. You've taken everything else, why not that, too?"

Kenton snorted. "I've taken nothing from you. You live like a queen."

The viscountess erupted in frenetic laughter, and Kenton's body went rigid.

His wife's green eyes glittered as if infected with madness. "You've taken everything that matters," she wailed. "My children can't abide you. You destroy whatever peace I manage to attain. And when I found a man who loved me, you ruined him."

Shock coursed through Anne. The wild-eyed, opium-affected viscountess appeared crazed, rationality gone along with all restraint.

"Have you no shame? Your lover was no more than a Lothario."

"He was a good man who dared to love me. While *you*," Lady Kenton added with revulsion, "are a *devil*." She used so much emphasis, spittle flew.

"Be quiet."

Anne heard more than a husband's command. A warning tolled in his voice.

"Why? I think Easterbrook has already discovered your secret." Lady Kenton pointed to the red, swollen crest of her cheek. "You hit. And you rape." She indicated Anne with a tip of her head. "*She* knows."

Anne expected escalating anger, but instead Kenton's face sagged into a kind of grimace. He squared his shoulders, the picture of a man overcome with grief and pain yet determined to be strong. "You're delusional." He looked at Peter. "I haven't wanted to admit it, but I can't deny her condition any longer. She belongs in a lunatic asylum."

Alarm chased across Peter's face. "But...she's intoxicated. Perhaps she's acquired an unhealthy compulsion, but surely commitment isn't necessary."

Lady Kenton directed her suddenly teary gaze to Peter. "I spoke the truth, so I'm to disappear into a hospital for lunatics?"

Kenton ignored his wife and spoke to Peter. "You can see she's become irrational, and I've seen the vicissitudes of her mind for some time."

The viscountess's eyes and mouth rounded in a look of pure horror. "*You're* the one who rapes and lies, and now my reward for years of silence is commitment in an asylum? No one comes out of those places!"

Kenton tipped his head back and stared at the ceiling as if beseeching God.

Lady Kenton squeezed the chair she still clung to and faced Peter. "I was here when he came home...after raping *her* mother."

She didn't look at Anne, but it was clear who the viscountess meant. Anne gasped. A slurry of ice rushed through her veins, while a deluge of sleet pricked her skin. Her gaze collided with Peter's. They stepped toward each other and clasped hands. The connection made tears swim into her eyes but she blinked them away.

"He said he'd been riding and a tree branch cut him." Kenton had snapped out of his reverie, real or performance, and Lady Kenton pointed to his facial scar. "No tree branch did *that*. That's from a rock, just like his victim said. His knees were muddy and grass-stained and there was blood where his trousers buttoned. There was bruising and swelling all around the cheek wound, and he was *livid*. There was no call for that."

"Enough of your raving, Claire," Kenton barked. He took a deep breath and looked to Peter. Shook his head and shrugged. "It's total invention. She's trying to strike back at me. It'd be best if you left. This is accomplishing nothing."

"Find his old valet and ask him," Lady Kenton urged. "Hopkins stitched the wound and cleaned the clothing stains. When Emma Albright cried rape, Hopkins knew the accusation was true. He could overlook a man disciplining his wife and children, but he had too much pride to be in service to a rapist. He left the same day."

"Why didn't he tell someone in authority?" Anne blurted.

"Hopkins received a generous bonus and a reference. They quieted his guilt. It would have been pointless anyway. He knew the word of a servant and a girl wouldn't stand against a viscount."

"Hopkins's corroboration might not have convinced an officer of the law, but it would have made a difference to my mother and the people who live here," Anne said. Peter gave her hand a squeeze, and her chest filled with warmth. Less than an hour ago, he'd vowed to learn the truth. Now he had it.

"I'm moving to the inn," Peter said. "Today. I can't stay here."

"You believe Claire's fabrications?" Kenton gave a laugh, as if the very idea were preposterous. "Don't you realize? If you won't take my word on this, you'll drive a breach between us, toss away the years I advised you in your father's stead. I may be guilty of being an authoritarian husband and father, but, Peter!" Kenton made an exasperated sound. "Have you asked yourself why I'd rape anyone? I'm wealthy, even-featured, and titled. You know yourself how attractive that makes a man. How it clouds women's judgment, how they can later regret their indiscretion."

Peter made no reply, and Kenton's incredulity disappeared. He closed his eyes and exhaled heavily, clearly disappointed. "Your father would be ashamed. Ashamed you've become such an...*ineffectual* man."

Anne's stomach churned. This was her father, and she hated him. She did.

Peter's voice emerged firm and sure. Nothing like how she felt. "I followed my father's example of manhood, and I've nothing to be ashamed of. I have the evidence of my own eyes that you abused your wife today. All these years, you hid your true nature from me. You're about to discover how far from ineffectual I am."

"You'll regret this," Kenton said. He turned and stalked from the room.

Trembling, Lady Kenton moved to the divan and sat. Peter gave Anne's hand another squeeze; then he released her and sat beside the viscountess.

"Let me take you to your daughter's. I can't endanger Arthur and his family by staying in their home, but they'd welcome you. You shouldn't remain here."

The viscountess nodded. She bent, reached under the hem of her skirt, and withdrew a laudanum bottle. Evidently she had a pocket in her petticoat. She pulled the cork and took a sip.

"Lady Kenton, would you consent to staying at my home?" Anne asked. "You need help. Perhaps my mother and I could be of assistance." Her resentment at the years of rebuffs had vanished in a moment.

The viscountess stared at the bottle, rubbing her thumb up and down the neck. She looked at Anne, hard, then ducked her head and gave a nod. After taking another sip, she corked the bottle and replaced it under her skirt.

Peter stood and began to move toward the door.

Anne followed.

"I'll ask the housekeeper to send someone to help you pack," he told Lady Kenton.

The group discovered Greggs standing at the top of the stairs. Peter put a staying hand on Anne's arm and said, "Greggs, tell Mr. Young that Miss Brown is to wait. She's not to leave until she speaks with me. He's to ask Mrs. Fairchild to send a different maid to Lady Kenton and order up a carriage. One big enough for four plus luggage. Then you can pack my belongings. All of them. I'm moving to the Fish Inn, as is Miss Brown. I'll see Lady Kenton and Miss Albright to their destination, too."

Greggs gave a short nod and hurried down the stairs.

"I'll make sure Miss Brown has money enough for a few days at the inn, the coach, and train fare," Peter assured Anne. "Plus a little extra."

"Thank you." Anne paused, hating saying this next thing, but she had to. "I'm happy you're leaving this household, but at the same time, I don't want you to. You may not be safe at the inn. You need to stay here."

"I can't." Peter shook his head and gave her an encouraging smile. "We don't think he's in the area anymore. I should be safe tonight."

"But what about after tonight? What if he comes back?"

"Broken bones or not, I have to leave Buttermere and go home. Tomorrow, if I can."

Anne's heart stopped. What about his promise to wait for her? But his life… Her eyes went hot, and she steeled herself. He was leaving for all the right reasons. She wanted him to live.

He smoothed a stray wisp of hair behind her ear. That brief touch made her yearn for his arms. Just one more embrace…

"I need to talk with Arthur before I go. Today, if possible. He and Belinda need to know what's happened. Given what her parents said, Belinda may have experienced strong and possibly even excessive discipline growing up. If so, she hid the truth from Arthur. He'll be devastated, but he needs to know. They also both need to know about Lady Kenton."

Anne nodded. Peter was right, and kind Mr. Jennett *would* be hurt. She thought the clergyman would be able to help, though, both his wife's and his mother-in-law's spiritual injuries. The law certainly wasn't on the women's side.

"Traveling such a distance will be painful," Anne warned.

Peter sighed. "I can make it to Treewick Hall. I'll be safe there while I figure out who's after me. Then, as soon as the criminal is apprehended, I'll be back."

A Roman candle of stars burst inside her. "You're coming back?"

His arm wrapped about her waist. He pulled her against him and kissed her. A long, powerful, thrilling kiss. One that made her heart fly about inside her chest. His mouth gentled, and their lips clung as the kiss ended, and then he said, "You need to get this straight. I love you. I'm committed to you. And I'll be back for you."

Anne took a breath that filled and spread her lungs. "Godspeed."

CHAPTER THIRTY-THREE

Two hours later, after delivering Lady Kenton and Anne to the Albright cottage and Rosella Brown to the Fish Inn, Peter knocked at Arthur and Belinda's door. He'd already spoken with Constable Weaver, who listened intently while Peter told him everything Lady Kenton had revealed. He approved of Peter's plan, and they agreed to stay in contact. Peter planned to stay the night at the Fish Inn and leave for home tomorrow.

Anne appeared to approve of his plan, too. He'd always remember how she looked when she wished him godspeed, her face and eyes glowing with love. When he returned he'd ask her—once again—to marry him.

The cottage door swung open. Belinda stood there, a silencing finger held to her lips. "Shhhhhh," she whispered. "The children are napping." Then she stepped back and waved him in.

Peter entered and waited while she eased the door closed. "Is Arthur here?" he asked softly. "I need to speak with both of you."

Belinda's brows rose. "He's in the study. Shall I bring tea?"

"I doubt we'd drink it," Peter said. Though he wouldn't turn down spirits if Arthur offered.

Belinda led the way. Arthur looked up, grinned, and stood when they entered.

"This is a pleasant surprise!"

His happy smile faded quickly. Arthur knew Peter better than anyone. He clearly saw this wasn't a social call.

"I've quite a lot to tell you," Peter said. "You need to be made aware."

He squinted against the light coming through the window behind Arthur's desk and motioned for Belinda to take one of the two empty chairs. Peter took the other, and Arthur sank into his desk chair.

"Have you discovered who's responsible for the attacks?" Arthur asked.

"No. This isn't to do with me." Peter couldn't think of a way to ease into his news, so he turned to Belinda and softened his voice. "Your father struck your mother today. Knocked her off her feet and bruised her face."

Expressionless, Belinda dropped her gaze to her interlocked hands. Arthur's mouth opened and he shot to his feet. Rounding his desk, he went to Belinda and crouched beside her. His hand covered his wife's, and he kissed her temple. Peter noticed she didn't unlock her fingers and take her husband's hand but kept them clutched together.

When Belinda didn't look at him, Arthur turned back to Peter. "Is she all right? Why didn't you bring her here?"

"She's at the Albrights' cottage."

Belinda's head shot up. "What is she doing there?"

"Anne was at Pennyton checking on me, and she got pulled into the situation. Lady Kenton was intoxicated. She's developed an unhealthy fondness for laudanum. I think you know, Belinda?"

Alarm flashed across Belinda's face, but she didn't speak.

"Anne offered to help, and your mother agreed it best she stay with the Albrights."

"Belinda? Did you know about this?" Arthur stopped and shook his head as if trying to align his thoughts.

"There's more," Peter said. "Perhaps you should bring your chair over here? This could take some time."

Arthur nodded. Peter's discomfort and sadness sat like a boulder in his belly as his cousin moved his desk chair and resettled himself.

"Some things your parents said made me wonder if your father had ever struck you? Or whipped you?" Peter said to Belinda. Arthur started to shake his head, but he stopped when he saw his wife's face. "With more force than should ever be used on a child?"

Belinda pressed her lips together.

"Perhaps even when punishment wasn't justified?"

Silence fell.

"Belinda?" Arthur whispered.

Belinda gave a little shake of her head and turned her face away.

"Belinda!"

Arthur sounded hurt as well as shocked. He shot Peter a wounded, questioning look, which Peter met and kept his own steady.

His cousin took a deep breath, leaned over and slipped an arm around his wife. For a moment she didn't move. Then her head turned back toward her husband and she sighed.

"Father has a quick temper. Sometimes he lashes out." She spoke with surprising matter-of-factness, and her husband stared in disbelief. What must Arthur feel, Peter wondered, to discover Belinda had hidden such a thing, apparently for years?

"I imagine this is something you don't like thinking about," Peter said.

Belinda gave a tiny shrug.

Arthur palmed his forehead. "Dear God in Heaven," he said. "How could I not know this?"

"Father's discipline may have been harsh, but I'm none the worse for it. There was no need for you to know."

"You grew up fearing your father? Of being hurt by him? Of course I should know."

Belinda gave an exasperated huff. "You were hurt and didn't understand when Father wouldn't consent to our marriage. His discipline practices would have been one more thing you didn't understand and felt bad about." They all heard Rebecca cry, and Belinda stood. "I need to go to the baby."

"I'm afraid I have more to tell you," Peter said.

"Tell Arthur. He can tell me later," Belinda replied, and she swept out of the room.

Arthur turned grim eyes to Peter. "What else?"

"Lady Kenton claimed her husband raped Emma Albright that night."

Arthur's mouth fell open. He dragged in a huge breath and whistled through pursed lips. "That's...unexpected."

"She rattled off some pretty convincing memories—details about the facial injury and blood at the opening of his trousers—and said Kenton's former valet, a man named Hopkins, could corroborate all of it. The valet resigned the day Emma claimed rape. Kenton maintained the viscountess invented everything, of course. He was calm, and she was stupefied and ranting."

"What do *you* think?"

What did Peter think? Lady Kenton's agitation had been spurred by opium and alcohol, but in spite of her impairment, Peter had seen sincerity and heard honesty. "I believe her. My mind is still reeling, trying to absorb it all."

Mouth tight, Arthur nodded.

"Arthur...Kenton threatened to commit her to a lunatic asylum. To shut her up."

Arthur bowed his head and covered his eyes. "Oh, Jesus."

Peter didn't take the utterance as a curse. These words were a call for help.

His cousin looked up. "To be so vile." His hand fisted and thumped his thigh. "He fooled me completely. I met him a few times when he came to Treewick Hall as your parents' guest, but I've really only known him six years, since my appointment as rector. Four of those years, he's been my father-in-law. And he's a pillar of this community. I haven't known him at all."

Peter nodded. He knew exactly how Arthur felt, because he felt the same: confused, betrayed, and guilty. He should have seen beneath the pretense. He ached for his cousin, who bore the additional burden of not realizing his wife carried painful secrets. She must have always been in need of her husband's care, but he hadn't known.

"Why didn't he want you for Belinda, exactly?" The son of a viscount's younger brother, Arthur was a usual sort of match for a viscount's daughter, and in Peter's opinion his cousin's character had no equal. Why would Kenton object?

"I wasn't grand enough." Arthur said.

"What do you mean?"

"He wants all his children connected to wealthy, socially prominent, powerful people. Belinda was the only one who didn't make an extremely advantageous match. You know them all, but perhaps you've never considered how far above their rank each married. Robert, the heir, married a much-sought-after duke's daughter, Amanda an earl, William found an heiress, and Mary outdid them all."

Peter had attended Mary's wedding. The woman was now a duchess.

"Kenton's offspring are attractive, intelligent, and admired," he said, "although I suppose no more so than many others. I assume the girls had substantial dowries?"

"Their dowries were average," Arthur said. "One brother or sister achieving an unexpectedly advantageous marriage wouldn't be noteworthy, but all? And Belinda was expected to marry a man with wealth or a title, too, but she fell in love with me."

"Expected. You say this because of the matches her brothers and sisters made?"

"No. She told me as much. Her father promised there would be a desirable prospect among her suitors, but she refused her London debut and insisted she'd never consider any other man but me. And Kenton relented."

"So easily?" Peter asked.

"Belinda didn't say it was easy," Arthur admitted. "But Kenton never showed me anything but gentility. Despite Belinda's assertion that our match spoiled his plans."

"You think he obtained superior mates for his children by placing them, or possibly their parents, under some sort of obligation?"

"I don't know, but my father-in-law has followed a lifelong practice of making influential friends and now counts some genuinely amazing men among them. He has an uncanny ability for fitting his mood and personality to the person he's with. I don't know it's so but, given he's a man with secrets, perhaps he's made a point of learning and trading other men's secrets? I believe he did so with Hewell, whom Amanda married, but that's the only match I'm privy to the details."

"Which are?"

"Hewell's title was good, but he needed money. He's obsessed with racing and likes to bet. Unfortunately, he has no talent for picking winners. He'd gotten deeply into debt. Then he bet everything on a slow horse with a huge handicap and unexpectedly won. There were nasty rumors a fast horse had been illegally substituted for the lookalike lollygagger. Hewell was suspected of having prior knowledge or somehow being involved. The Jockey Club was investigating. Kenton stepped in, dispelled fellow Jockey Club members' suspicions, and quieted the rumors. *Somehow* Hewell had money enough to pay his debts *and* buy a couple winning Pennyton racers. Kenton sponsored him when he applied for Jockey Club membership. Fortune and reputation repaired, a short time later Hewell married Amanda."

"If Kenton's playing men against their secrets, he's taking a risk of becoming embroiled in scandal. Why would he do that? Not for financial gain. He has plenty."

"For privilege, power, and a legacy, I suppose. None of which I enhance."

A sudden thought struck with power enough to cleave Peter's brain in half. Stunned, he froze while his mind shot in a hundred different directions. Had he gone mad? He hated giving voice to the idea, but its plausibility grew with each passing second until it became a soul-deep certainty that would not be denied.

Arthur watched with attentive eyes. His cousin knew him, had deduced something was wrong and was waiting.

"Could Kenton be...the one who wants me dead? You and Belinda would then be Lord and Lady Easterbrook. You'd inherit my properties and all my wealth."

Air burst from Arthur like he'd been punched in the belly. He steepled his hands over his nose and mouth and bent forward as if in pain. He and Peter stared at each other a long time. Finally, Arthur straightened and lowered his hands. "I can't refute it. Not now that we know what his duplicity has hidden all these years."

A harsh laugh erupted from Peter's chest. "If Kenton is the one, it explains why the trap didn't work. He helped plan it. He knew all would think the culprit had left the area and relax. Once everyone's guard dropped, I'd be easier to get to. Thank God Lady Kenton opened my eyes."

"I've shared meals and holidays with him, worshipped with him, prayed with him at my wedding and babies' christenings. Suddenly I discover he's a monster." Arthur's voice carried bleakness coupled with despair.

Peter thought about his recent conversations with Kenton. "A monster who's smart, makes excuses, and believes himself right-minded. That makes him especially dangerous, and means he won't give up."

Arthur rubbed his temples. "To think I encouraged Belinda to forgive her father for withholding his blessing when we wanted to wed. I've been so blind." He grimaced. "Now I must explain her father's a rapist and, assuming Owen Weaver's death can be laid at his door, a murderer. How do I tell her?"

"You love her. The words will come." Peter stood. "She already knows her father's a monster. She may not be surprised to learn his evil is even darker than she knew. Her childhood mistreatment may be harder for her to discuss."

Arthur got to his feet, moving like he'd aged thirty years. When Peter embraced him, his cousin returned the hug with an extra measure of pressure.

They broke apart. "If it is Kenton trying to kill me, he's paying the attacker. The wisest thing is for me to go home. I'd already planned to leave tomorrow, so no one will be surprised. I'll be safe at Treewick Hall, and when the assassin makes another attempt, we'll get him. If he names Kenton as the man who hired him, we'll have evidence. I'll write, keep you informed. You do the same."

"Of course." Arthur's brow creased. "How will you go? Tomorrow's not a day the coach runs."

"While I was in the village talking to Constable Weaver, Richard Thorpe came by checking for news. Tomorrow's his half day and he's visiting a lady friend in Borrowdale. He offered to drive me on to Keswick. I'll catch the coach there. Red can remain in Snow's care until I send a groom for him."

"I'm happy to hear Thorpe has a lady friend. Before I wed Belinda, she confessed that she and Thorpe once shared a romantic attachment. I've always suspected he never quite got over her."

"I remember your jealousy," Peter said. "But now we know that was silly. Did Kenton know? I can't imagine him permitting such an association. Not with Thorpe's father being Kenton's stable master. And Thorpe has always worked for Kenton." Thinking of how his godfather would have reacted to an adolescent Belinda consorting with a servant made Peter cringe.

"No one knew. They were riding companions as children, and as they grew up they continued to ride together almost daily. No one thought twice about their spending time together."

"I wonder if Thorpe ever suspected Kenton of abusing Belinda or other family members? When you talk with her, ask if that's something she wants others to know. Everyone's going to find out Emma told the truth. Learning Kenton also abused his family could change the attitude of those residents who never fully accepted Belinda."

"I'll ask."

"I hope to make a quick return. I'm anxious to put this behind me and make plans for the future. I hope to have you officiate at my wedding before the year is out."

A slow smile curved Arthur's mouth. "Your wedding to Anne. Nothing would please me more."

CHAPTER THIRTY-FOUR

They were between Buttermere and Borrowdale, the lake on Peter's right, the fell to his left, when the carriage stopped. Peter looked out and saw a gate in the stone wall that ran along the road. The gate was closed, and all was quiet. The problem could be anything, he supposed—a horse, harness, or the road itself.

He didn't have long to wait before Richard Thorpe opened the door. Leaning against the carriage with one raised arm, the horse breeder glanced up and down the road before addressing Peter. "Let me help you down. I need to drive off the road to get past this, and it'll be too bumpy for your broken bones. You'd best walk around."

"What's the problem?"

Seeming distracted, Thorpe gazed up and down Honister Pass. "A wagon with a broken wheel. The owner went for help or supplies, I suppose. Some of the load spilled, and the road's completely blocked."

In his mind, Peter groaned. Climbing in and out of the carriage was hell on his ribs, but he supposed it was far better than jolting about while the carriage crossed rough ground. He was cradling his ribs and stepping down when something bashed his head and obliterated the world.

~

Anne dismounted, secured Snowflake, and strolled among the trees. Dressing Thomas Russell's surgical wound had been her last task of the day. Edwin would be happy to learn that the farmer was healing well from his toe amputation.

She needed to supplement her dwindling supply of angelica, and Crag Wood, a good spot to find wild angelica, was on her way home. There was still plenty of light. While looking for the plant's tall, umbrella-like clusters of tiny white flowers, she enjoyed the sounds of birds, the rustle of leaves in the trees, and the view of Buttermere's blue water. The jumble of emotions she'd experienced yesterday had exhausted her, making her appreciate the wood's loveliness even more than usual.

How long would it be until she received Peter's first letter? A buzz of warm excitement spread down the back of her neck and over her shoulders. She'd never received a letter that included words of love, but she knew she could expect them from him with another proposal of marriage. She couldn't wait.

She wondered how Peter's talk with Mr. Jennett had gone. Quite different than the one she had with her mum, she guessed. Thinking of Mum's face when Anne described yesterday's events and revelations, Anne couldn't help but smile. Vindication, after twenty-four years. Once they'd discussed all that occurred in Lady Kenton's sitting room, Anne had explained she was finding her way to forgiving Peter his secrets and missteps. Smiling, her eyes warm and happy, Mum had hugged her and hurried to Edwin's.

Movement in the corner of Anne's eye drew her attention to the water. Through the trees she glimpsed a man and woman standing beside a beached rowboat. Their raised voices carried, but not well enough to make out the words. Large, emphatic gestures added to Anne's impression they were arguing.

The woman turned her head, and Anne froze. Could that be Belinda? Anne appraised the man with increased interest. Not the rector, she was certain of that. This man had a broader, more powerful frame than Arthur Jennett. Feeling a bit guilty for what could be construed as spying, Anne still moved closer.

Her stomach swooped into her throat.

The man looked like Thorpe, but Richard Thorpe was supposed to be driving Peter to Keswick. He shouldn't be here, arguing with Belinda. Unless...had Peter's plans changed?

Anne continued navigating through the trees, closing the distance. A few more yards and she'd be able to make out their words. A soft whicker drew her attention away from the shore, and tucked away behind a thick clump of trees, hidden from the road by foliage and shadows, was a carriage and horses. A mare with a sidesaddle waited beside them.

Hurrying to the carriage, Anne threw open the door. Empty. Was Peter here? She scanned the quiet wood. Should she call out to Belinda and Thorpe? An uneasy *something* kept her quiet and made her approach them covertly, tree-to-tree, in a clandestine manner.

Suddenly, Belinda's voice became distinct. "All right, have it your way. So let's push off. I'm here to help, just as you wanted, but I don't have much time. I've got to get back to Rebecca. She'll need to nurse."

Anne stopped behind a tree large enough to hide her and peered around its trunk.

"This is our best opportunity." Belinda's voice lost its impatient edge and became persuasive. "If you can't do it right here, right now as we planned, then this will give you a little time. You can put something over his head and he won't know it's coming. Then you can make it look like you were ambushed and Easterbrook was kidnapped. His body can be found later."

All Anne's breath left her lungs and tears sprang in her eyes. Fear unlike anything she'd ever known surged through her veins. She dug her nails into her concealing tree's bark. Where was Peter?

Thorpe looked across the water. "Maybe we could dump him in when we get to the middle? Just leave him and row away. By the time we get back to shore, it'll be over."

Belinda was shaking her head before he finished. "In order for him to be declared dead and Arthur to inherit, there's got to be a body. Now, let's go."

He was alive. Hope lifted Anne, and she scanned the shoreline and wood again. Where was he?

Thorpe hesitated a moment then offered Belinda his hand. She stepped into the boat and suddenly Anne caught an unobstructed view of the stern and the crumpled form lying on the bottom. Peter! It had to be Peter!

They were taking him across the lake. Aside from fells, there was nothing over there but trees, pasture, and sheep.

She needed a weapon. What could she do without one except be caught and overpowered by Thorpe? Anne ran back toward Snowflake and the pistol she kept in her saddlebag. Thorpe would be moving to the bow, shoving off. He'd have to turn the boat. She might have enough time. She had to hurry.

Nothing existed but pumping legs and heaving lungs, urgency and her will. She reached Snowflake and seconds later was racing back, pistol gripped in her hand. Her lungs burned. She kept running, but a few moments later got a clear look through the trees.

They were already out in the lake! He'd turned the boat and they were yards away, heading toward the opposite shore. Thorpe rowed with a fast, powerful stroke, creating a white bloom where the bow cut the water. Spray flew from the ends of the oars each time they lifted. It took hard rowing to get that kind of speed and breaking water. They were flying.

What should she do? Constable Weaver was in Buttermere. There wasn't time to fetch him. She'd go around the lake and meet them on the other side. Surprise them. Pray they didn't do what Thorpe suggested and simply dump him in the water. But Belinda had suggested there was some other plan.

A minute later, Anne and Snowflake were out of the trees and headed south at a gallop, making a wide arc with Gatesgarth Farm at its apex. As much as she wanted to take the shortest route, along the shoreline, Anne couldn't. There weren't any trees along the southern part of the lake. If she followed the shore, Belinda and Thorpe would probably see her. Right now, surprise was her single advantage. If only they hadn't gotten a head start on her.

A short while later the stone buildings of the sheep farm came into view. Thank God. She left the road, sent Snowflake over the low stone wall, and pulled her up between the barn and the house.

"Mr. Marshall!" Anne yelled. On her third shout of his name, Marshall's wife rushed from the house.

"Miss Albright. What's wrong? Gilbert's in town." Mrs. Marshall hurried to Snowflake's heaving side.

"Fetch the constable. Tell him 'Easterbrook's assailant is Richard Thorpe.' Tell him to come to the west side of the lake as fast as he can. I think Thorpe's headed to the midpoint or lower."

Wide-eyed, Mrs. Marshall gathered up the skirt of her apron and clenched and twisted the fabric. Four children of various ages came out of the house and clustered together. Anne knew them all. Thank goodness the oldest girl was of an age to mind the younger children.

"Mrs. Marshall," Anne snapped. "Did you hear? Do you understand? A man's life is at stake." Snowflake sensed her tension and sidled. "Take your fastest horse. Please, hurry."

Anne's gravity and commanding tone must have gotten through, because Mrs. Marshall nodded. "I'll go immediately."

Anne pointed Snowflake at the wall. "Be careful," Mrs. Marshall called as they sailed over.

Anne headed for the west side of the lake. Once she reached woods again, she'd follow the trail. Belinda and Thorpe's boat was too far away to make out details, but it had either stopped or was moving slow. They should have been across by now. Maybe Thorpe had gotten tired. Whatever the reason, it gave Anne more time.
Thank God.

Be alive, Peter. I'm coming.

CHAPTER THIRTY-FIVE

Peter awoke gagged and trussed in the stern of a rowboat. He lay on his side, against the bottom planks. Facing him, Thorpe rowed. A cloaked woman sat between them, her back to Peter.

Pain and comprehension struck together. Thorpe worked for Kenton. *Thorpe* was the paid assassin, the man who'd murdered Owen, who'd shot and assaulted Peter. Christ, the pain in his head was excruciating, and he couldn't pull his thoughts together. His sling hung from his neck, empty. His broken arm was *behind* him, his wrists tied together. Where the break was, Peter's arm burned like the devil's hand encircled it, a murderous grip squeezing hard. Peter's legs were bound at the ankles. His coat pocket didn't have the bulge and weight it should have. Most likely Thorpe had taken his pistol.

He tried to sit up. His head whirled and throbbed so hard that his mind faded for a bit. Once that cleared, a constant, muffled whine assaulted his ears. A vise crushed his head.

He forced his limbs to relax, told himself to wait, breathe, and not panic. Some of the haze cleared. This time he moved nothing but his head, adjusting its position in small increments so his mind wouldn't revolt.

"He's awake," Thorpe said.

The woman looked over her shoulder.

No! God, no! *Belinda*!

For a moment his pain, his restraints, *everything* was gone. Relief and amusement buzzed through him. He was asleep, suspended in a nightmare, nothing more. Then the physical world returned, and with it, suffocating despair. This was real.

How had Belinda come to be here? Was her presence some sort of demented punishment meted out by her father? Perhaps Kenton intended Belinda's guilt, knowing Peter died as a sort of gift for her, to provide him with a means of control? Peter tried to dislodge the gag and talk to her, but it seemed glued to the insides of his mouth. Anger pervaded every part of him. Anger so extreme, he thought he might dissipate into bloody mist. He gagged, coughed, discovered his air passage blocked, and went still. Forced himself to calm and breathe slowly through his nose.

Belinda! If she were harmed, Arthur would be devastated. Thank God Thorpe hadn't restrained her. There was hope she could somehow get the best of Thorpe or get Peter free.

"This should all be over and done with," Belinda said. "It's been more than two months!"

Peter went cold. What did she mean? She couldn't mean—

"It's not so easy to kill a man in cold blood." Thorpe's words sounded boiled-out-of-a-kettle hot.

"I suppose I know that, since the only killing you've accomplished was done in self-defense. Even that wouldn't have happened if I hadn't been there distracting Weaver."

She spoke to Thorpe as if they were...in collusion.

Thorpe scowled. "If I believed you meant to keep your promises, I'd be more determined."

"You'll be paid once Arthur inherits. Enough for your own stud farm."

Thorpe's eyes narrowed. "I don't give a damn about the money. You know I'm doing this for *us*, not a stud farm."

Horror cocooned Peter and squeezed tighter than his bonds.

Belinda and Thorpe were working together. Belinda—not Kenton—wanted him dead.

"I know my happiness means everything to you." Belinda swept the hood of her cloak off her head. "We have to finish this. There's no other way I can settle my children's lives, give them the lives they're meant to have. I can't make it happen without you."

Thorpe had almost stopped pulling the oars. Their emotions were high, they were entirely focused on each other. It was Peter's best chance.

One after the other, he tried to draw up his leg and wriggle his foot free of the fetters. Like the rope encircling his wrists, the one around his ankles was wrapped tight. He bent his knees, arched his back, and moving slow, slow, slow tried to get his feet high enough behind him so his hand could reach the knot. If his hands would even work. They'd both gone numb. He strained hard, as high as he could bear.

It was no use. He went limp and breathed.

Thorpe stopped rowing and rested his forearms on his thighs. "What about *our* lives, Belinda? Doing this is supposed to lead to a different life for *us*. One we share. You said you want that as much as I do."

"You said you'd be patient with me," was her rejoinder. "Instead you're making demands. I've been beset with nervousness since we began this... this..." She waved her hand in a gesture of vexation. "Pursuit. Your dissatisfaction with me and your four—no, five—bungled attempts to dispatch Peter haven't helped." She gave a sharp laugh. "My father destroys lives and apparently his conscience is guilt free. I've become a wreck."

Thorpe's hands fisted. "I'm expected to have endless patience, am I? You forget I've waited years. Years you dedicated to *him*."

She turned her head, gazed at the water, and Peter saw Belinda's chin quiver. A moment later her mouth firmed and she turned back to face her accomplice.

"I thought, when I married Arthur, I was escaping. No more punishment from Father, no more dead babies. No more *fear*!"

A wave of shock slammed through Peter. *Dead babies?* What did that mean? Had Belinda borne and lost a baby before her marriage? Her arms moved; he knew she wiped tears from her cheeks.

"If we'd eloped, you'd have had nothing to fear," Thorpe said. "Not your father, not Hell. You'd be—" He stopped, made a choking noise. "You'd be sinless, and our sweet babe would be alive."

Horror descended on Peter like a beast of a storm—black, full of electricity, sucking away the very air he breathed. Thorpe couldn't mean, *he couldn't mean…*

"You refused to understand, but I thought Arthur would save me," she said, voice wavering. "I thought I'd find absolution through his goodness, by following his example. I've tried my best, but being his wife didn't work. The guilt weighs as heavy as it ever did, and now I have children cursed with this way of life. You want assurances, but until this business with Peter is finished and my children's futures are secured, I can't think about myself."

Peter's stunned mind whirled. Arthur had confided worries about his wife's psyche, and dear God, but it sounded like his concern was justified. It was too little, in fact. Arthur had never suggested he suspected infidelity, yet how else could Peter interpret Belinda and Thorpe's exchange? He wished he could see her face.

Thorpe lifted the oars from the rowlocks and laid them along the sides of the boat.

"Why are you stopping?" Belinda asked. "Are your hands cramping?"

Thorpe's head dropped. He sat with eyes closed, hands interlocked and pressed to his mouth.

"Richard? Do you want me to row?"

The horseman straightened, blowing out a long stream of air through pursed lips. "I can't kill him—Easterbrook."

Belinda gasped. The boat rocked a bit in the ripples caused by the breeze. "You can't back out now."

Thorpe swung his head back and forth in denial. The corners of his mouth drooped. "I never should have agreed. I wanted you, and you convinced me it would be simple, but it's not simple! It's a terrible, cold-blooded act." He extended shaking, spread-fingered hands toward her. "You think you're nervous? Look at me." He sounded as if he blamed her for his state. "I'm shaking, and sweating, and my heart is pounding. It never stops." He pressed his hand to his chest. "If you truly cared about me, our future wouldn't be dependent on my committing murder for you. I've already killed one good man. I don't want to kill a second."

"Yes, you've killed a man," Belinda said, her voice fierce, "and now you *have* to kill Peter. He's right here, seeing and hearing everything!" She threw up her hands. "Every moment we're out here, we risk being seen. We can't sit here and dither. Don't you realize? The money comes through him.

"You say you love me. So, *help* me. That's what you do when you love someone. The way Arthur *tried* to help me. The way I *am* going to help my children. You're *keeping* the promise you made."

Thorpe's eyes went dark, his mouth twisted. "You don't believe I love you?"

Belinda emitted a shrill bark of amusement. "You'll forget me once you have your own stud farm. You'll be a prosperous bachelor who'll appeal to many women. But until then, be sensible and row!"

Thorpe's lips parted and his eyes went wide. "You were never doing it for us. It was always for *him*. Arthur." He gave a harsh laugh. "Do you know, I had my own plan, before I discovered how distasteful killing is? After dealing with Peter Jennett, I intended to kill your husband and leave your *son* Lord Easterbrook. With your husband gone, there'd be nothing to keep us apart."

Belinda sprang to her feet, and the small boat rocked. She wobbled, spread her arms away from her sides and balanced. Alarm flashed across Richard's face. He slowly rose.

"Sit down, before you tip us over," he warned.

"Kill Arthur? How could you imagine I'd condone you killing Arthur? Did you think I'd forgive you and welcome you with open arms? You're mad."

"Yes," he shouted. "That's exactly what I thought. You said, together we'd create a bright, new future, and I was fool enough to believe you.

I reasoned, why not go one step further? We'd be free to marry and have all the riches as well.

"Remember the day young Weaver happened upon us and discovered the truth? I never would have bested him if I'd been alone. He was a soldier. Proficient at a soldier's business and steady. Except, he underestimated you. His attention was on me, and *you* leaped on him. He lost his gun, and I got lucky."

"*You* killed him."

"Yes, I did. With your help. Afterward, I wondered if you'd been using me all along. Whenever I balked, you were ready with assurance and affection." Thorpe jerked his cap off, swiped his forehead with his arm. "I succumbed again, less than an hour ago," he said with a tone of bewilderment, "but the row across Buttermere gave me a chance to think. So many promises, embraces, kisses, yet I've never felt passion from you. Not for years. It was all a sham, wasn't it?"

"You know you were the first man I loved. My feelings for you go deep." At her sides, her hands clenched into fists. "We'll both be happy, Richard. After you kill Peter."

But Thorpe's face was that of a rejected suitor, not a welcomed one. "Perhaps, if I want to make sure it all concludes the way you've promised, I should kill Arthur first and do away with Peter after."

Belinda shrieked, surged forward, and thumped his chest with her fists.

Thorpe pushed her away. His broken laugh was that of a disillusioned man. "I've turned the tables, haven't I?"

She charged, leapt, and cannoned into him, hard. The boat rocked violently. A look of alarm and surprise swept Thorpe's face, and he spread his arms in a wild, blind grab at air. He fell back and his head hit the gunwale with a crack, the boat gave a ferocious heave and tilted Belinda off-balance. Arms wheeling, she tried to keep her feet as the vessel rocked wildly. She stumbled, her body tipped sideways, and her legs rammed against the hard edge of the boat. With a startled cry, she toppled into the cold water of Buttermere.

Peter threw his shoulders and rolled up to his knees with a heave and an involuntary cry of pain. He couldn't stand or crawl, but kneeling he could see the water. There was no sign of Belinda.

Thorpe lay crumpled in the bow, unconscious.

Belinda's head broke the surface, and one hand grabbed at the air. Wet hair streamed over her face. "Rich—" she choked out. And went down.

She didn't swim! Helplessness and fear exploded in Peter. Angling his back to the side of the boat and moving his knees the small amount his bonds permitted, he got his wrists atop the gunwale. Maybe he could loosen the rope or the knot. Using only his right arm, the injured left forced to move along, he sawed the rope back and forth against the edge. His throat worked in a soundless cry. The stabbing pain in his broken arm was too great... He stopped. Oh, God. God, no. He couldn't give up! He had to get free!

He tried again. A few saws and his vision went dark. Tiny bright lights flew before his eyes like a spray of embers. He stopped and let his arms fall from the gunwale. Sweat trickled down his forehead, into his eye. The rope hadn't loosened.

Several yards from the boat, Belinda's head broke the surface again. It bobbed there, and she sputtered, coughed. Head tilted back, she stretched her neck...and went under mid gasp.

Peter opened his mouth as wide as he could, tried to work his tongue, and heaved in air through his nose. The wad of cloth, stuffed firmly inside his mouth, didn't move. His jaw barely moved, but he worked it the small amount he could and tried to move his tongue. He gagged. He relaxed his throat, breathed. Tried again, with the same result. Each time he attempted to move his tongue, the reflex at the back of his throat clenched and he retched. The runaway pounding of his heart spread from his chest to his head.

The gag moved! He sucked in air, pushed, pushed, pushed his tongue, retching each time. The gag moved again. Just a little. Just enough to get his tongue working. And then the wad shifted. He pushed it out and gulped air.

Belinda rose again, coughing, choking. Her hand emerged, grasping for something that wasn't there.

Peter called out; nothing but a raspy squawk emerged.

His tongue hurt and seemed to fill his mouth. He tried to cough, wet his mouth, swallow. Her head bobbed down…up, and he got a clear look at her terror. Neck stretched, head tilted, only her eyes and nose were above the water. She sputtered, made choking noises.

"Float on your back," he managed to call out, but his voice didn't sound normal. Could she hear him? He wasn't sure. Her eyes had gone glassy, unfocused. He filled his lungs, yelled as best as he could. "Go limp. Float on your back. Kick your feet."

She cried out, the noise little more than a croak, but Peter understood the brief vocalization. Arthur's name.

She sank…and didn't come up again.

CHAPTER THIRTY-SIX

Long minutes passed. Peter stared at the spot where Belinda disappeared until all hope faded.

He lifted his gaze from the calm blue water to the sky and the craggy green hills around him. A complex mix of emotions churned in his chest. Foremost among them was sadness for Arthur, little Henry and Rebecca, and for the horrifying turn Belinda's life had taken. Other emotions buffeted, keeping him off balance and confused. It would be a while before he sorted it all out.

Thorpe moaned, opened his eyes, and sat up rubbing the back of his head. His palm came away bloody and he swiped it against his trousers.

"Belinda drowned. She lost her balance and toppled out."

All signs of pain disappeared from Thorpe's face, replaced by horror. He surged up and wildly scanned the lake. Dropped to the bench and started to remove a boot.

"It's no use," Peter said. "It's been too long. She's gone."

Thorpe's face crumpled; his shoulders bent. He buried his face in his hands and his shoulders shook.

Moving his knees by small degrees, Peter traversed to the bench Belinda had occupied. He managed to seat himself, lift his legs, and swing about to face Thorpe. Then he waited. The man seemed to be calming, taking a couple deep breaths.

Thorpe lowered his hands from wet, red-rimmed eyes. "She didn't swim. When we were children, the boys all learned but the girls didn't." He closed his eyes. "I loved her," he explained, voice thin and scratchy. "I always loved her." He looked at Peter. His mouth went tight and his eyes flashed. "You bloody bastard. Why are you so hard to kill?"

Peter kept his voice low and steady. "Let's go back to the horses."

"And then what? I turn myself in? Or have an hour's head start before you're found and the constabulary is after me?"

Thorpe picked up the oars and rowed—toward the west side of the lake, away from the horses and Honister Pass. He didn't speak, and Peter kept silent. Thorpe seemed in a hurry, and once across let the boat glide toward the shore and beach. He hopped out and pulled the boat farther ashore, then sprang back in and moved to Peter. Before Peter realized what the man intended, he'd dragged Peter to the end of the bench.

"Stand up," Thorpe ordered.

The man steadied Peter as Peter stood, then his captor swung himself over the side. He put his shoulder to Peter's middle, his arm between his legs, grabbed under Peter's arm and hoisted him across his shoulder. Peter cried out, the pain of Thorpe's shoulder pressing against his fractured ribs overwhelming every other thought and feeling. Peter panted, held as still as he could.

"Don't fall off," Thorpe warned. "You won't like what happens if you do."

The man navigated through a hundred yards of close-spaced pine trees before reaching open ground. The lake now obscured by trees, Peter saw a tall hill and grassland populated with Herdwick sheep. A rocky stream ran down the hillside above them and a number of rough-textured granite boulders lay scattered about. A small rock shelter sat a distance away.

Thorpe carried him through the shelter's doorless entry and dropped him to the dirt floor. Luckily Peter's back and right side took the impact; the landing hurt, but the pang passed. It was a shepherd's hut, a crude structure intended to provide shelter from lightning and weather. Hope rose that Thorpe was going to leave him here, eventually to be found by a shepherd, hunter, or someone taking a constitutional walk.

The horseman drew a pistol from his pocket.

Peter's hope crashed, and a grimmer purpose occurred. Thorpe meant for the hut to hide Peter's dead body.

"Leave me here. It could be days before I'm found. You can be well away, somewhere on the Continent. Even bound for America or Australia."

"Change my name, forfeit my reputation as one of the best steeplechase breeders and trainers in the country? I think not."

"You're not a killer. You told Belinda you couldn't kill me."

Like an animal caught in a trap, Thorpe's eyes glittered wildly. "Belinda's *gone*. Gone, believing I didn't love her. If I'd just *killed* you, everything would be fine." The hinge of the man's jaw bulged. His lips drew back, exposing clamped teeth. "I'm not going to hang. I'm going to live, and I'm going to give her children the future she planned."

Thorpe raised the pistol. It wobbled.

"Don't do it, Richard. You'll spend the rest of your life running from yourself."

Thorpe adjusted and tightened his grip. "You're wrong. My qualms are gone. Your mystery killer is going to succeed. I can attest to being stopped on the road by a masked man and hit on the head. I have the scalp wound to prove it." He rubbed the back of his head. "Belinda's horse will be found, and Belinda will be missing." He dragged in a breath through his nose. "I suppose it'll be assumed she became another unfortunate victim, in the wrong place at the wrong time."

"Don't you want her to have a proper burial? I can tell them what occurred, and her body will be retrieved. You're a resourceful man. You'll find your way and build your reputation again."

Thorpe seemed to think it over. His mouth turned down. "I'd like that, but it's better that I don't leave."

The sound of a galloping horse reached them. Thorpe whirled and ran outside.

Who was coming? Whoever it was, he'd ride straight into Thorpe's ambush. The rider's only chance of a warning was Peter, and also Peter's only hope of rescue, so he braced for the pain and rolled to his back. A giant vise clenched his arm between its jaws and squeezed. He gritted his teeth. Bent his knees. Pushed with his feet and scooted toward the door. He focused his mind on the doorway and *moving*, and breathed, pushed, scooted. He did it again, and again, until his head lay in the doorway. The hoofbeats were close.

Peter unlocked his aching jaw, filled his lungs, and as a horse burst into his field of view, yelled, "Ambush!"

Everything seemed to happen at once. The identity of the horse—Snowflake—and the rider—Anne—registered at the same moment Anne reined in hard and a pistol barked. Snowflake screamed, forelegs lifting off the ground, head and body twisting. Anne came off the mare's back and hit the ground. She still wore her medical bag slung across her body.

Peter's heart lodged in his throat, still racing. A narrow wound scored the mare's neck; the bullet had creased her.

Anne scrambled up in a flurry of skirt and grabbed Snowflake's reins. The horse, agitatedly dancing, settled a bit. Anne lunged for the saddlebag.

What was she doing? "Run!"

Fifteen yards away, Thorpe exploded from behind a bush and sprinted toward Anne full tilt. He'd shot his round, he'd want to nab her.

Anne!

She unbuckled the saddlebag with a couple jerks and reached in. Thorpe was nearly there.

Please, God, help her!

Anne pulled out a pistol, dropped the reins, and using both hands leveled and cocked the gun. Ten feet away, Thorpe planted his feet and braced, stopping abruptly.

"Don't move."

Any other woman would be hysterical, Peter believed, but not Anne. He heard tension in her voice, but she was as calm and collected as an officer of the law. A blast of love shot through his chest. Strength flowed into his limbs and his pain eased.

Except, Thorpe *did* move. He slid a hand into his coat pocket, withdrew a different pistol, and aimed it at Anne. Peter recognized the firearm. It had started today's journey in his coat pocket.

"Thorpe! For God's sake, man! Not Anne. You can't."

Anne started, and her gaze flew to Peter. Some of the tension smoothed from her face.

"Are you all right?" she called.

"I'm in fine fettle," he assured her. "The very best."

Anne nodded.

Peter hardened his voice. "Thorpe… Think, man. Kill us, and there'll be too many dead. You'll fall under suspicion. Weaver'll leave no stone unturned. You know that. Get away. Now, while you can."

Thorpe's jaw worked. No sound came out. Then came the sound of sudden hoofbeats from the north.

"That's the constable," Anne said, her voice ringing with certainty. "And he knows it was you."

Thorpe ran toward the lake and disappeared into the trees. Anne looked at Peter, then in Thorpe's direction.

"Leave him to Weaver," Peter said.

Anne ran to him and dropped to her knees. She was there. So beautiful, with tears suddenly spilling from her eyes.

"Thank God," she said, voice shaking. "Thank God. I was so afraid you were dead." She gave him a short, hard kiss, bent around behind him, and tugged at the knot behind his back.

"Easy, love." Peter grinned. He couldn't help it.

She sniffed and opened the medical bag at her hip. Held up a pair of shears. Using small snips, she worked at the rope and a moment later Peter's hands were free. Pain bit his fingers and palms at the return of circulation.

"Let me," she said.

Slow and gentle, she moved his fractured arm to his side, bent the elbow and positioned his forearm across his chest. His sling still hung around his neck, and she slipped his arm inside. The relief was immense and immediate. With the limb in its natural position and supported, much of his pain resolved. He released a huge sigh.

Anne cradled his face and kissed him. It was, perhaps, the best kiss of his life. For a moment, everything in his world was perfect.

They parted and smiled at each other, and inside, the sun rose.

"Your feet," she said, and moved to release the rope around his ankles.

The galloping horse was near. The constable, Peter hoped. Just like Anne had claimed.

"Here!" Anne called.

A moment later the constable reined his mount up near Snowflake.

"He's got a boat." Peter pointed toward the lake, where they'd beached.

"Thorpe's the one?" Weaver asked.

"Yes," Peter said. "And he killed Owen."

Weaver made a noise that sounded like a vocalization of pain. He dismounted, pulled an Enfield from the sleeve attached to his saddle, and headed into the trees.

Anne pulled the last of the rope from Peter's ankles. She helped him kneel then stand. Being on his feet with his limbs free felt liberating. He took her hand and they followed after Weaver.

They found the constable with boot toes nudging the water's edge, rifle-musket trained on Thorpe. Rowing hard, the horseman was halfway across the lake—an easy reach for a good shot with one of the new Enfields.

"Thorpe, stop," Weaver called. "I've got you in my sights. I'll shoot if I must."

Thorpe's only response was to bend lower and row harder.

"Last chance," Weaver called. "Turn the boat around."

Thorpe stopped rowing, raised his pistol, and fired. The shot went wide, not unexpected for a handgun at that distance. Weaver's steady aim didn't budge. But he also didn't fire.

Thorpe picked up the oars and resumed rowing toward the east shore. Facing west as he pulled, he stared straight at Weaver. The Enfield cracked, and smoke bloomed from the barrel. Hit in the chest, Thorpe dropped the oars and folded.

No one spoke. Breeze-generated waves lapped the shore.

"I couldn't let him get away," Weaver said. He faced Peter and Anne. "That boat he's in is mine, the one I keep on the east shore. I'll ride to Gatesgarth Farm. They'll have a boat I can use, and Marshall will give me a hand."

"Belinda Jennett's body is in the lake," Peter said. "I saw her drown. It was an accident, but she was behind everything."

Weaver appeared to think that over and gave a nod. "Do you intend to tell Mr. Jennett? Or should I?"

"I'll tell him," Peter said. Arthur should hear the news from him.

"There's a carriage and three horses across the lake in Crag Wood," Anne said.

Weaver's gaze swept Peter. "Do you need help getting back?"

Peter held out his hand to Anne. "I think Snowflake can carry us both. We'll keep to a walk."

They returned to the stone hut and collected the mare. Weaver headed his bay toward Gatesgarth Farm.

After delivering a few loving words and rubs to Snowflake Anne mounted, and Peter swung up behind her. Once settled, he wrapped his arms around her waist. She leaned back a little and rested lightly against him.

"Does this hurt?" she asked.

"I'm fine." The pressure of her body didn't hurt, but he still had a lot of healing to do. In addition to the physical pain, helping Arthur through his grief and remorse would be heart-rending.

Anne gave a nod and signaled Snowflake, who started walking. Peter tightened his arms, pressed himself against Anne's back, kissed the side of her neck. Then he said something that was surprisingly true.

"Right now, the only thing I feel is happy."

EPILOGUE

Three years later

Anne sat on the divan in Treewick Hall's library, her two-year-old Julia on one side of her and Rebecca on the other. They paged through Rebecca's picture book, while Henry played nearby with his collie, Samson.

Peter had created the dearly-loved book using sketches and water-colors of places and people familiar to Rebecca. Among others there was a drawing of her rocking horse, looking much more alive than the one in her bedroom; Anne and Peter standing under Henry's tree-house holding the children's hands; and one of Anne's favorites, a tottery one-year-old Julia hugging Samson. Anne turned the page to a scene from her mother's wedding to Edwin.

"There you are scattering flower petals in the church, Rebecca. Remember?"

Rebecca nodded. "Petals from Grandmother Kenton's garden."

Lady Kenton now lived year-round at Pennyton Park, happily estranged from her husband. Kenton had escaped ill will and ugly gossip by going to the Continent, but if Anne ever happened to face him again, she knew she could and still keep her head.

Peter called her name and walked in, smiling broadly and waving a letter. Excitement fairly radiated from him. The children looked up.

"Is it news about the Manchester Assize Court commission?" she asked. The architectural design he'd submitted was under consideration.

"No." Peter glanced from Anne to Henry. "It's news from Arthur."

Henry's happy look faded and an all too familiar solemn expression took its place. The boy stopped his tug-of-war with Samson and got up from the floor.

Peter sat across from Anne and the girls. Henry moved closer and placed his hand on Samson's head. Anne put her arm around Rebecca's shoulders and gave the girl a quick hug. It would be good news, Anne felt sure. Peter looked too happy for it to be otherwise.

"He's coming home." Simple words, but Peter spoke them as if they proved God's benevolence.

Rebecca gave a glad cry, clapped, and bounced a few times.

Happiness swept through Anne. "Wonderful!" They'd waited and hoped for Arthur's return for three long years.

Henry didn't move; his set, frowning expression didn't change. "For a visit? Or for good?"

Peter lifted the page. "Let me read it." He leaned back against the chair, raised the letter, and began.

"'To my dear children, Henry and Rebecca; my cousins, Peter and Anne; and my newest little cousin, Julia. Greetings, dearest family. I've resigned my post with the Church Mission Society and plan to leave India in two weeks. Barring any complications, I expect to reach England by January first." Peter looked up. "Perhaps in time for your birthday, Henry."

"Or even Christmas," Anne added.

Henry didn't remark. Did Arthur realize he was coming home to a son who still had nightmares about his father's abandonment, and a daughter who didn't remember him?

Peter continued. "'I'm familiarizing my replacement with his teaching duties, and trying to contain my eagerness to see you all. For now, I have no plans beyond my arrival home. I've decided to delay accepting a position until after I've reacquainted myself with my children, and they with me.'"

Miss Tangent, the children's nanny, came to the door.

"Excuse me, my lord, my lady. Please forgive the interruption. I promised the children we'd visit the kittens in the stable this afternoon."

The children all perked up, and the girls slid down from the divan.

"May we?" Henry asked, eager as Samson when offered a scrap.

"Certainly. I was nearly finished, anyway." Peter folded the letter and slipped it in his pocket. "He closes by sending his love."

Miss Tangent held out her hands, and the girls ran to her. Henry and Samson followed them out.

Peter crossed to the door and closed it, then returned to the divan and sat beside Anne. He indicated the picture book still open on her lap.

"I need to add a couple drawings, don't you think? It's been a while."

"Perhaps the kittens?"

"Good idea."

She closed the book and set it aside. His eyes gleamed, their corners crinkled a little, and he leaned close. Anticipation fluttered in her belly.

He kissed her, and Anne kissed him back—gladly, lovingly, and even a touch lustfully.

When their lips parted, Peter pressed his forehead to hers. "You fill my heart to overflowing, do you know that?"

Anne's chest filled with a warmth as grand and remarkable as life itself. "I have a reservoir of love to draw from, and I promise it won't run dry."

Peter drew back a few inches. "I remember how amazed I was when you insisted we forgo our wedding trip to settle Henry and Rebecca. You didn't hesitate."

"Not for a minute. It hurt so much, knowing what Belinda tried to do, but I had no trouble loving her children."

"I'll never forget how certain you were. I was thunderstruck, and I worried I wouldn't be the guardian they needed. You were not only willing but confident we'd be worthy foster parents. You never doubted my ability to give the love and reassurance they needed. I'm so glad we expanded our family, new as it was. As much as I gave, I received tenfold back."

"I'm grateful Arthur has healed enough to come home. You know, he and the children will need our help." The thought made Anne's chest go soft, while her spine went stiff. The coming days would be challenging and emotional. She would help any way she could.

"And once they adjust, they'll leave and we'll be lonely. Especially Julia."

"Well..." Happiness filled her heart, heat singed her cheeks, and Anne's hand went to her belly. Was this the time to tell him?

"Well...what? You don't agree?"

Given his general look of confusion, Peter was baffled. Anne took his hand. "She shouldn't be too lonely, given we'll soon be a family of four."

Peter gave a shout, grabbed her, and wrapped her in joy. For a moment she marveled at how love, and Peter, had changed her. She remained a nurse who was frequently called upon, but in addition had the very different and wonderful and sometimes exasperating experiences of a beloved wife and mother. Anne pulled away, gazed into eyes brimming with love, and knew she looked straight into his heart—nothing hidden, nothing held back. "I didn't think I could hold more happiness, yet somehow my gladness never seems to stop growing."

As if he couldn't bear not to, Peter pressed a quick kiss to her lips. "Every time I decide it can't get better, it does. I was afraid you'd be resentful I'd made you part of the aristocracy, but I know you aren't."

"I'm proud to be your viscountess. If one day I find myself the mother of a future Viscount Easterbrook, I'll be bursting."

So much behind her, so much ahead. What an adventure her future held: the wonder, love, and joy of a lifetime with Peter. She loved every bone in her husband's body—especially the mended ones.

AUTHOR'S NOTE

Thank you for reading *Never a Viscount*. I hope you enjoyed it.

As with all my books, my medical characters employ treatments that were readily available in 1856 England, and at least somewhat effective. Thorn-apple was smoked as an asthma treatment for centuries, and both thorn-apple and caffeine have a mild bronchodilation effect.

I thought it likely Peter's gunshot wound would become infected, and before the advent of antibiotics, simple infections could progress and become fatal. I wondered if it were possible for a person to survive sepsis, known in the nineteenth century as pyemia or suppurative fever. Civil War medical reports state the rate of mortality from pyemia as ninety-seven percent. This was pyemia from all types of infections, not just wounds. While survival of pyemia prior to the era of antibiotics was apparently possible, it was most commonly felt to be one to two percent.

Luckily I came across the Astley Cooper prize essay for 1868, *On Pyemia or Suppurative Fever*, by Peter Murray Braidwood, MD, publisher John Churchill & Sons, London. Dr. Braidwood collected data on suppurative fever throughout his career. Of the twenty suppurative fever patients he treated, only one—a twelve-year-old boy—survived. Dr. Braidwood kept detailed notes on the different types of suppurative fever, its four different, progressive stages, and the length of each stage. The course of the illness was long, with the final recuperative stage of convalescence lasting around thirty days. If it seems as though Peter is sick an extraordinarily long time, it's because I made the course and length of his disease as accurate as I could.

The idea for the racetrack scheme Arthur's brother-in-law is associated with came from my reading about a racetrack grifter named Peter Christian Barrie. Working first in England, then moving to the U.S. in the 1920s, Barrie perpetrated a horse "painting" or "ringing" scam using bleach, ammonia, adhesive bandages, silver nitrate, henna, and exotic dyes. He would bleach, then dye a fast racehorse to give it the exact appearance of a slow runner, and switch the two. Expert at transforming a horse's looks, he could achieve any number of effects including dappling and white markings. He even plucked tail hairs, arranged manes, and drilled teeth to achieve an identical match. Horses' jockeys, trainers, and owners were fooled to such an extent, they'd swear the substitute was their horse. Switch accomplished, Barrie bet on the replacement, which ran with the long odds of the lookalike slow horse. The horse would win and Barrie would make a bundle. The con was in making everyone think the (slow) winner simply had an incredibly good day.

In 1851, Buttermere's population was a mere seventy-eight. It's a beautiful spot but must have been very remote. There was a nearby slate mine that employed many Buttermere residents, with the slate transported out across the mountains by pack horse. Today the main industry is sheep farming, and Herdwick sheep roam the Lake District. A local breed of Norse pedigree, Herdwicks are born mostly black and lighten with age.

Thanks again and happy reading!

ACKNOWLEDGMENTS

My sincere thanks:

This book has been so long in the making, seeming to hit one "life roadblock" after another, until it became almost humorous. It passed through several phases and several generous friends who lent their critique skills to different drafts. To Carrie Padgett and Bethany Goble, not only for critiquing the last two drafts, but for the encouragement that kept me going. I am soooo thankful you hung in there with me. To JoAnn Sky, whose advise helped shape the first draft. And to Patricia Heineman for her input through the early drafts. Thank you, my friends, thank you.

And to editor Chris Keeslar for his story guidance and editing finesse. It was a long haul but… we did it!

OTHER BOOKS BY SHERI HUMPHREYS

A Hero to Hold

The Nightingales Series

The Unseducible Earl

By the Light of a Christmas Moon (an Unseducible Earl spinoff)

The Seduction of Cameron MacKay

Anthologies

Rescued

You'll find them all at:

Amazon

iBooks

Barnes & Noble

Rakuten kobo

You might also enjoy reading

Mustcat Tales

a free serialized story of an audacious winery cat

Sign up to be notified of Sheri's new releases here

ABOUT THE AUTHOR

Sheri Humphreys used to be an Emergency Room nurse, but today applies bandages, splints, and slings to the characters of her Victorian romance novels. Her book, A Hero to Hold, received a prized Kirkus Star and was named to Kirkus Reviews' Best Books of 2016. She lives with Mama Catt, a mouser of renown, in a small town on the central California coast.

Visit her home on the web! http://sherihumphreys.com

Made in the USA
Monee, IL
09 February 2022